VOLUME 2

Cellular and Molecular Mechanisms of Inflammation

Vascular Adhesion Molecules

VOLUME 2

Cellular and Molecular Mechanisms of Inflammation

Vascular Adhesion Molecules

Edited by

Charles G. Cochrane
Department of Immunology
Research Institute of Scripps Clinic
La Jolla, California

Michael A. Gimbrone, Jr.
Department of Pathology
Brigham and Women's Hospital
Harvard Medical School
Boston, Massachusetts

Academic Press, Inc.
Harcourt Brace Jovanovich, Publishers
San Diego New York Boston London Sydney Tokyo Toronto

This book is printed on acid-free paper. ♾

Academic Press, Inc.
San Diego, California 92101

United Kingdom Edition published by
Academic Press Limited
24–28 Oval Road, London NW1 7DX

International Standard Serial Number: 1052-5882

International Standard Book Number: 0-12-150402-6

PRINTED IN THE UNITED STATES OF AMERICA
91 92 93 94 9 8 7 6 5 4 3 2 1

Table of Contents

Preface

The localized attachment of circulating leukocytes to the lining of small blood vessels long has been recognized as the cellular hallmark of the inflammatory response. This adhesive interaction, a necessary antecedent to the emigration of leukocytes into tissues, traditionally has been viewed as a manifestation of the leukocyte-directed action of chemoattractant stimuli. Nonetheless, more than a century ago, Cohnheim suggested that molecular changes in the vascular lining might be involved. This notion, that the luminal surface of the endothelium might become locally hyper-adhesive, has become a recent focus of intensive investigation and fast-paced discovery.

This volume of *Cellular and Molecular Mechanisms of Inflammation* addresses the rapidly expanding field of vascular adhesion molecules. It reviews our current understanding of the structure and function of constitutive and inducible cell surface structures, which contribute to the temporal and spatial patterns, and cellular selectivity of leukocyte–vessel wall interactions. These include the recently described SELECTINS (or LEC-CAMS), a family of structurally related glycoproteins that contain lectin like domains that confer leukocyte-selective adhesive functions. ELAM-1, induced in vascular endothelial cells by cytokines and bacterial endotoxin, primarily supports the attachment of neutrophils and certain lymphocytes, while GMP-140 (PADGEM, CD62), a granule membrane-associated protein transiently expressed at the endothelial (and platelet) surface in response to rapid agonists such as thrombin, appears to interact with neutrophils and monocytes. The third member of this family, LAM-1 (gp 90^{mel}, LEC-CAM-1, LECAM-1), has long been recognized as a homing receptor directing the traffic of subsets of lymphocytes through the high endothelial venules of lymphoid organs. More recently, this and analogous leukocyte surface molecules have been found also to interact with vascular addressins, counter-receptors in inflamed tissues. A common denominator of the SELECTINS is their use of carbohydrate-based recognition mechanisms involving various cell surface components. Yet other adhesive molecules, such as CD44, may recognize glycosaminoglycans associated with extracellular matrix. Also considered are members of the immunoglobulin family of cell surface glycoprotiens, including ICAM-1 (CD54), VCAM-1/INCAM-110, which interact with various heterodimeric integrin receptors (e.g., LFA-1, Mac-1, VLA-4) present on leukocytes; and LPAM-1, a novel integrin type lymphocyte homing receptor.

In keeping with the philosophy of this series, we have asked active investigators to contribute their perspective on a selected aspect of this complex field. While this approach may not yield a comprehensive picture, hopefully the contents of this volume will prove informative and stimulating to those interested in the cellular and molecular mechanisms of inflammation.

M. A. Gimbrone, Jr.
C. G. Cochrane

CHAPTER 1

Endothelial-Leukocyte Adhesion Molecule-1 (ELAM-1): A Vascular SELECTIN That Regulates Inflammation

M.P. Bevilacqua, C. Corless, and S.K. Lo

Vascular Research Division
Department of Pathology
Brigham and Women's Hospital and
Harvard Medical School
Boston, Massachusetts 02115

1. Introduction

Cell–cell recognition and adhesion are key events in biological processes ranging from fertilization to immunological defense. The field of vascular biology has witnessed explosive interest in the mechanisms and molecules involved in inflammation. In 1980, endothelial cells were not known to express specific adhesion molecules for circulating blood cells, nor did the dominant theories of inflammation require them. One decade later, a total of five endothelial-leukocyte adhesion molecules thought to participate in

Cellular and Molecular Mechanisms of Inflammation, Volume 2

inflammatory adhesion events had been identified, cloned, and characterized (Fig. 1). Two of these molecules, endothelial-leukocyte adhesion molecule-1 (ELAM-1) (this chapter) and granular membrane protein-140 (GMP-140; also called PADGEM or CD62) (Johnston *et al.*, 1989; Chapter 2), are members of a new family referred to as vascular SELECTINS (Bevilacqua, 1989) (Table I) or LECCAMS (Stoolman, 1989). The third member of the SELECTIN family, the murine MEL-14 lymph node homing receptor (mLHR) (Siegelman *et al.*, 1989; Lasky *et al.*, 1989), is expressed on neutrophils, monocytes, and most lymphocytes, as is its human counterpart leukocyte adhesion molecule-1 (LAM-1 also known as Leu8 or TQ1) (Tedder *et al.*, 1989; Camerini *et al.*, 1989; Chapter 3). Each of the vascular SELECTINS is thought to play an important role in the interaction of blood cells with endothelium. Three other cell adhesion molecules on endothelial cells that support leukocyte adhesion are members of the immunoglobulin gene superfamily. These are intercellular adhesion molecule-1 (ICAM-1), intercellular adhesion molecule-2 (ICAM-2), and inducible cell adhesion molecule-110 (INCAM-110), also known as vascular cell adhesion molecule-1 (VCAM-1). The pattern of expression of these five endothelial molecules as well as their target cell selectivity appear to be important factors in the regulation of leukocyte sequestration and trafficking across endothelium during inflammatory events.

This chapter will focus on ELAM-1, a cytokine inducible endothelial molecule that supports the binding of blood neutrophils, monocytes, and a subpopulation of lymphocytes *in vitro*. It is designed less as a comprehensive review of the field than as a perspective on an interesting mol-

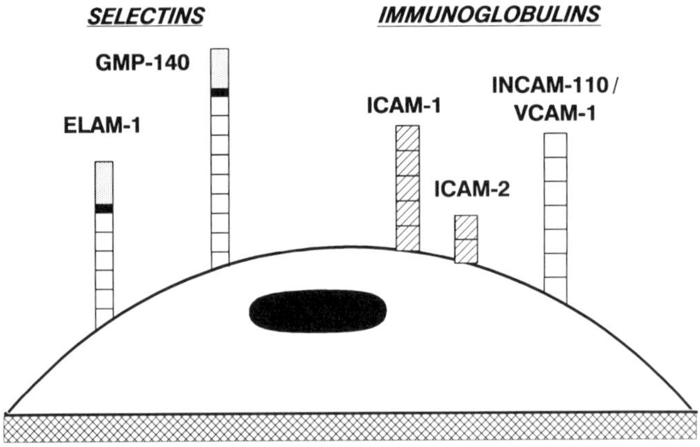

FIGURE 1

Endothelial-leukocyte adhesion molecules.

TABLE I

Vascular SELECTINS

Molecule	Expressed by	Binds
ELAM-1	Endothelium (activated)	PMN, mono, few lymph
GMP-140/PADGEM	Endothelium, platelets	PMN, mono
mLHR/LAM-1	Lymph, PMN, mono	LN-HEV, endothelium (activated)

ecule. As part of this perspective, ELAM-1 will be compared to the other SELECTINS; for now, we would like to highlight one common feature of these molecules, namely the N-terminal domain of each SELECTIN, which contains a structural motif previously found in carbohydrate binding proteins (C-type lectins; Drickamer, 1988). A variety of complex carbohydrates are coupled to cell surface proteins and lipids. These carbohydrates have tremendous potential for containing biological information because they vary not only in the sequence of their monomeric units, but also in the position, anomeric configuration (α or β), and branching of these units (Sharon and Lis, 1989). In recognition of this structural diversity a role for carbohydrates in cell–cell recognition has long been proposed. The structural characterization of the SELECTINS led to the prediction that they bind carbohydrates, prompting intense and exciting research at the boundary of two fields, *cell adhesion* and *glycobiology.* A first fruit of this effort has been the demonstration by several laboratories that one or more of a related group of carbohydrates comprised of fucosylated lactosaminoglycans found on leukocytes and certain tumor cells can bind to the SELECTINS ELAM-1 and GMP-140.

II. ELAM-1 Structure and the SELECTIN Gene Family

Molecular cloning of ELAM-1 was undertaken using a complementary DNA (cDNA) library constructed with mRNA from cultured umbilical vein endothelial cells that had been treated with recombinant IL-1β (Bevilacqua *et al.*, 1989). This library was transfected into COS cells and a cDNA was isolated that encoded a cell surface molecule reactive with the anti-ELAM-1 antibodies H18/7 and H4/18. Furthermore, COS cells transfected with the ELAM-1 cDNA supported the adhesion of blood neutrophils. The translated sequence of the ELAM-1 cDNA predicted a polypeptide of 610 amino acids that includes a 21 amino acid signal peptide and has features consistent with a type 1 transmembrane protein. The extracellular region of ELAM-1 was divided into three segments based on homologies to previously described molecules. The aminoterminal region (approximately 120 amino acids) is related to several members of the C-type lectin family (Drickamer, 1988) that includes the low affinity IgE receptor (CD23), the asialo-glycoprotein receptor and the mannose binding protein. The lectin-like domain is followed by an epidermal growth factor (EGF) motif similar to that found in a variety of proteins. The ELAM-1 protein also contains six tandem nonidentical repeats (approximately 60 amino acids) that are structurally related to those found in a family of complement regulatory proteins. This family includes cell surface molecules such as complement receptors type 1 and 2, as well as the serum glycoproteins C4 binding protein and factor H. Several members of this family are known to bind complement factors C3b and C4b. To date, ELAM-1 has not been shown to bind complement components.

The unusual mosaic structure of ELAM-1 is shared by the cell adhesion molecules GMP-140 and mLHR/LAM-1 (Fig. 2). GMP-140, also called PADGEM, is a 140 kD transmembrane protein stored in granule compartments of platelets and endothelial cells (McEver *et al.*, 1989; Bonfanti *et al.*, 1989) (See Chapter 2). In these cell types, GMP-140 can be rapidly redistributed to the cell surface following stimulation by a variety of mediators including thrombin and histamine. The mLHR was identified with mAb Mel-14 as a murine lymphocyte cell surface structure involved in the homing of lymphocytes to peripheral lymph nodes (Gallatin *et al.*, 1983). Subsequent studies demonstrated that this molecule is also expressed on blood neutrophils and monocytes where it may play a role in acute inflammatory events (Lewinsohn *et al.*, 1987; Chapter 3). Cloning of GMP-140, as well as the mLHR and its human counterpart LAM-1, revealed structures similar to that of ELAM-1 (See Chapters 2 and 3). Each of these molecules contains an aminoterminal lectin-like domain, an EGF repeat, and multiple complement regulatory repeats. The coincident cloning of these structurally related molecules resulted in the birth of the new gene family termed vascular SELECTINS (Bevilacqua, 1989). The lectin-like and EGF motifs amongst members of vascular SELECTINS are greater than 60% identical at the amino acid level. There is approximately 40% identity within the complement regulatory repeats. Interestingly, each of the complement regulatory repeats of the SELECTINS contains six cysteines, a feature not shared by other known molecules with complement regulatory motifs, which contain only four cysteines. The number of complement regulatory repeats in the SELECTINS varies with GMP-140 having nine, ELAM-1 six, and the mLHR and LAM-1 two each.

Genomic clones encoding each of the vascular SELECTINS have been isolated and the organization of the genes has been determined. The

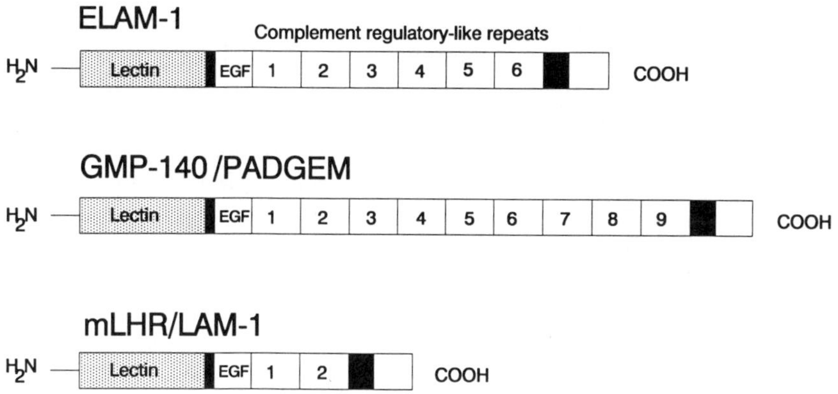

FIGURE 2
Domain-structure of vascular SELECTINS.

ELAM-1 gene, which is present in a single copy in the human genome, consists of 14 exons spanning about 13 kilobases of DNA (Collins *et al.*, 1991). The positions of exon-intron boundaries correlate with the putative functional subdivisions of the protein. Introns are found in similar positions in all of the six complement regulatory repeats suggesting that these elements arose by gene duplication. Similar structural organizations have been found for the gene of GMP-140 (See Chapter 2) and mLHR/LAM-1 (See Chapter 3). Moreover, gene linkage analysis in the mouse has indicated that these genes all map to a distal region of the mouse chromosome 1. Long range restriction site mapping showed that the genes were located within 300 kilobases in human and mouse genomes (Watson *et al.*, 1990). Together, these data suggest that the SELECTIN family may have arisen by multiple gene duplication events. It is also interesting that the location of these genes on chromosome 1 suggests an evolutionary relationship to the complement binding gene family members that are on the same chromosome and have substantial sequence homology (Watson *et al.*, 1990).

III. Sialyl Lewis X, A Carbohydrate Ligand for ELAM-1

The presence of a lectinlike domain at the amino terminus of ELAM-1 strongly suggested that this molecule may recognize a carbohydrate structure on blood leukocytes. This hypothesis gained support by the demonstration that the epitope recognized by the adhesion blocking monoclonal antibody H18/7 is located within the lectin domain in ELAM-1, with a contribution (possibly conformational) from the EGF repeat (Walz *et al.*, 1990). In contrast, the nonblocking antiELAM-1 mAb H4/18 binds within the first three complement regulatory-like repeats. Several laboratories have presented evidence showing that ELAM-1 and GMP-140 can interact with one or more members of a group of oligosaccharides comprised of fucosylated lactosamines (Fig. 3). Adhesion to ELAM-1 was found to correlate with the presence of the sialyl Lewis X antigen (sialyl CD15) on various leukocytes and tumor cell lines (Walz *et al.*, 1990; Lowe *et al.*, 1990). This correlation was substantiated by the finding that expression of a (α1,3)-fucosyl transferase in transfected cells generated surface fucosylated polylactosamines, including sialyl Lewis X, that supported adhesion of the cells to ELAM-1 (Lowe *et al.*, 1990). Further studies using monoclonal antibodies, as well as sialyl Lewis X bearing proteins and liposomes (Walz *et al.*, 1990; Phillips *et al.*, 1990) have provided additional evidence for an adhesive interaction between ELAM-1 and this carbohydrate structure. A direct approach to identification of ELAM-1 ligands was taken by Tiemeyer *et al.* (1991), who demonstrated that COS cells transfected with a cDNA encoding ELAM-1 adhere to a subset of sialylated glycolipids resolved on thin layer chromatography plates or absorbed on plastic. Structural analysis of the glycolipids that supported ELAM-1 dependent adhesion revealed sialylated lactosyl-ceramides with variable numbers of

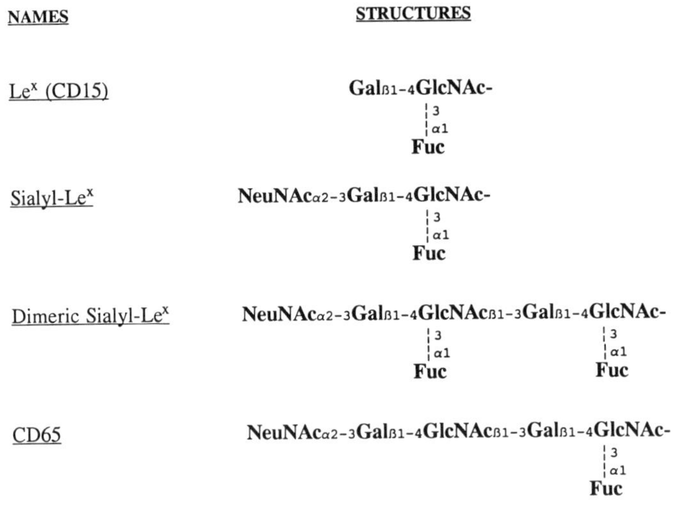

FIGURE 3

Structures of fucosyl-lactosaminoglycans.

N-acetyllactosamine repeats and at least one fucosylated N-acetylglucosamine. These investigators also showed that elimination of N-acetylneuraminic acid from the glycolipids abolished adhesion of ELAM-1. In summary, these studies strongly suggest that sialyl Lewis X and the related fucosylated N-acetyllactosamines found on leukocyte glycolipids and glycoproteins may act as ligands for ELAM-1.

The structural similarity within the SELECTIN family suggests that GMP-140 and mLHR/LAM-1 may recognize similar carbohydrate structures. Interestingly, Larsen *et al.* (1990) provided evidence that the non-sialylated structure of Lewis X (CD15) formed part of a ligand for GMP-140/PADGEM. Other studies have suggested that an α1-6 linked N-acetylneuraminic acid residue is important in GMP-140 mediated cell adhesion (Corral *et al.*, 1990; Moore *et al.*, 1991). The complete structure of the GMP-140 ligand(s) remains to be resolved. Carbohydrate ligands for mLHR/LAM-1 have yet to be identified, however, it is interesting to note that mLHR mediated adhesion is blocked by a number of negatively charged mono- and polysaccharides and by fucoidin, which is rich in fucose (Imai *et al.*, 1990). It is possible that fucose and N-acetylneuraminic acid are also important elements of mLHR ligands.

IV. Expression of ELAM-1 *in Vitro* and *in Vivo*

In Vitro systems have been utilized to study the expression of cell adhesion molecules on vascular endothelium. The five known endothelial-leukocyte adhesion molecules demonstrate distinct patterns of expression. ELAM-1 is not expressed on unstimulated human endothelial cells in culture. Consistent with a role for ELAM-1 in inflammation, exposure of endothelial monolayers to the cytokines IL-1 or TNF or to bacterial endotoxin results in a time- and protein synthesis-dependent expression of this glycoprotein (Bevilacqua *et al.*, 1987). Cell surface expression is detected within an hour after exposure to these inflammatory signals, reaches a peak level between 4 and 6 hours and subsequently declines toward baseline by 24 to 48 hours (Fig. 4). Expression of ELAM-1 mRNA transcripts in cultured endothelial cells was also shown to be induced by IL-1 and TNF, with a maximum at 2 to 4 hours and decay by 24 hours (Bevilacqua *et al.*, 1989).

Like ELAM-1, two other endothelial adhesion molecules, INCAM-110/VCAM-1 and ICAM-1, are also cytokine-inducible. In both cases, their expression is induced more slowly than that of ELAM-1, peaking at 8 to 24 hours (Fig. 4). In addition, INCAM-110/VCAM-1 and ICAM-1 expression

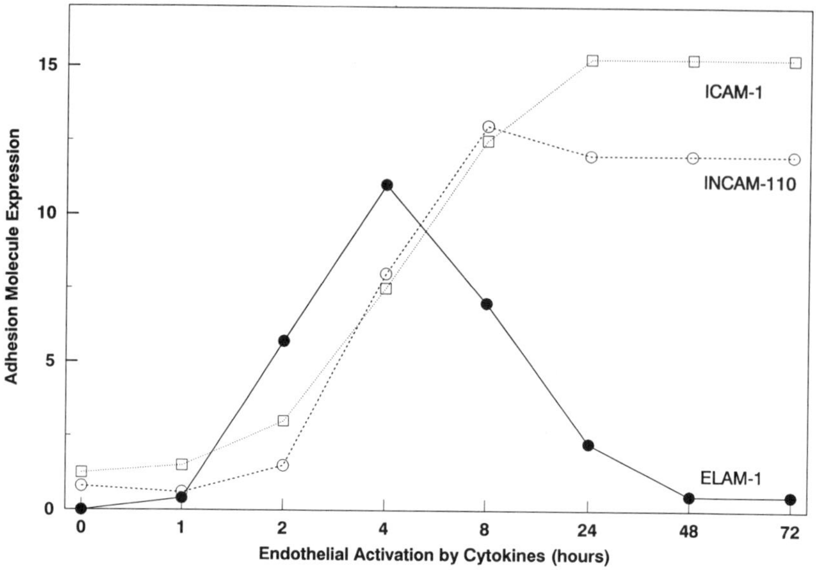

FIGURE 4

Temporal expression of endothelial adhesion molecules.

remains elevated for 72 hours or longer (Rice and Bevilacqua, 1989). Endothelial INCAM-110/VCAM-1 has been shown to support the adhesion of blood lymphocytes and monocytes (Osborn *et al.*, 1989; Rice *et al.*, 1990) through an interaction with the $\alpha^4\beta_1$ integrin (Elices *et al.*, 1990). INCAM-110/VCAM-1 does not appear to mediate neutrophil adhesion. ICAM-1 interacts with leukocyte beta-2 integrin CD11a/CD18 that is found on all leukocyte types (Marlin and Springer, 1987; Simmons *et al.*, 1988). Less is known about the expression of ICAM-2, which also binds CD11a/CD18; however, it has been demonstrated that the mRNA encoding this molecule is not affected by cytokines (Staunton *et al.*, 1989). GMP-140, the other endothelial SELECTIN, has its own unique pattern of expression. After synthesis, GMP-140 is stored as a transmembrane protein in Weibel-Palade bodies (See Chapter 2). Stimulation of endothelial cells with several mediators including thrombin and histamine (but not IL-1 or TNF) causes an immediate translocation of GMP-140 to the endothelial cell surface where it can support the adhesion of neutrophils (Geng *et al.*, 1990).

Studies of ELAM-1 function have demonstrated that this molecule can support the adhesion of neutrophils and monocytes, which correlates well with the high levels of expression of sialyl Lewis X on these leukocytes. It has been suggested that ELAM-1 can support the adhesion of memory T lymphocytes (Shimizu *et al.*, 1991) and a population of skin-homing memory lymphocytes (Picker *et al.*, 1991). To date, a lymphocyte cell surface structure recognized by ELAM-1 has not been described, but it appears that sialyl Lewis X is expressed on too small fraction of lymphocytes to account for all lymphocyte adhesion.

It has been suggested that the regulated expression of these adhesion molecules on endothelium *in vivo* may be a key factor in dictating the extrasvasation of selected leukocytes at sites of inflammation (reviewed in Pober and Cotran, 1991). Immunohistochemical studies of human tissues from a variety of disease states show ELAM-1 expression on vascular endothelium, preferentially in postcapillary venules (Cotran *et al.*, 1986). Strong expression of ELAM-1 has been reported in cases of appendicitis and other inflammatory disease processes involving substantial neutrophil infiltration. Studies with a baboon model demonstrated the temporal expression of ELAM-1 in inflammatory skin tissues induced by local injection of TNF (Munro *et al.*, 1989). ELAM-1 expression was detected within 2 hours of treatment and correlated with the influx of neutrophils. However, in human tissues ELAM-1 expression has also been observed in several pathophysiological states marked by an absence of neutrophil accumulation, including dermal delayed-type hypersensitivity and rheumatoid arthritis (Cotran *et al.*, 1986; Koch *et al.*, 1991). These data suggest that several factors may act together to regulate leukocyte extravasation.

Efforts to demonstrate the sialyl Lewis X antigen in inflammatory tissues revealed colocalization of ELAM-1 on endothelial cells and its ligand on leukocytes within the vessel and in the tissues. For example, in acute appendicitis, endothelium expressed ELAM-1 and adherent or emigrating leukocytes stained positive for sialyl Lewis X (Munro and Bevilacqua, manuscript in preparation).

V. Sialyl-Lewis X on Tumor Cells

Rice *et al.* (1988) observed the binding of melanoma cells to cytokine-activated endothelial cells and subsequently identified INCAM-110 as the major endothelial molecule involved in this adhesion (Rice and Bevilacqua, 1989). Taichman *et al.* (1991) have since determined that, like lymphocytes, melanoma cells bind to INCAM-110 through the $\alpha^4\beta_1$ integrin. It has also been demonstrated that HT-29 human colon carcinoma cells bind to activated endothelial cells (Dejana *et al.*, 1988), however, in this case, adhesion was shown to depend on ELAM-1 and not INCAM-110 (Rice and Bevilacqua, 1989). These observations suggested that tumors of different origin may interact with different classes of endothelial adhesion molecules.

The observation that HT-29 colon carcinoma cells bind to ELAM-1 suggested that the surface carbohydrates of these tumor cells might overlap with those of normal neutrophils. Interestingly, this overlap had already been noted in earlier studies by investigators working with anticarbohydrate monoclonal antibodies generated against carcinoma cells. Several of the antibodies cross-reacted with granulocytes, including anti-Lewis X and antisialyl Lewis X antibodies (Fukushima *et al.*, 1984; Symington *et al.*, 1985; Fukushi *et al.*, 1985). The relationship between expression of Lewis X related structures on tumor cells and binding to ELAM-1 has been examined (Walz *et al.*, 1990; Corless and Bevilacqua, unpublished observations). Of four human colon carcinoma cells lines examined, three showed ELAM-1 dependent adhesion to IL-1β activated endothelial cells, and all three reacted with an antisialyl Lewis X antibody (CSLEX1). A fourth cell line that expressed Lewis X but not sialyl Lewis X showed no adhesion to ELAM-1. Thus, like neutrophils, tumor cells appear to interact with ELAM-1 through surface sialyl Lewis X, although a contribution from related structures has not been excluded.

On nonleukocyte cell populations sialyl Lewis X is considered an oncofetal antigen. It is present on a variety of human carcinomas, particularly adenocarcinomas of the pancreas, colon, stomach, and lung but is rare in normal tissues, being detected only in renal tubular epithelium, esophageal glands, and occasional colonic crypts (Fukushima *et al.*, 1984; Fukushi *et al.*, 1985). The fetal intestine is rich in sialyl Lewis X (Fukushi *et al.*, 1985), as is amniotic fluid (Hanisch *et al.*, 1988), suggesting a role for this carbohydrate structure during fetal development. Elevated levels of sialyl Lewis X bearing molecules are detectable in the serum of many cancer patients (Chia *et al.*, 1985; Hirota *et al.*, 1985), and it has been proposed that sialyl Lewis X could serve as marker of tumor burden. Interestingly, sialyl Lewis X is present on carcinoembryonic antigen (CEA) (Chandrasekaran *et al.*, 1983); since CEA is shed by tumors into the bloodstream it is possible that it may bind to ELAM-1 at sites of inflammation and thereby inhibit inflammatory responses.

The expression of sialyl Lewis X on neutrophils and tumor cells is dependent on several glycosyltransferases, which are responsible for the synthesis of the underlying type II N-acetyllactosamine chain (Galβ1-4GlcNAcβ1-3Gal), terminal sialylation through an α2-3 linkage, and the addition of fucose to N-acetylglucosamine (see Fig. 3). The latter appears to be the key regulatory step (Holmes *et al.*, 1986), and in this light it is interesting that neutrophils and colon carcinoma cells appear to utilize different fucosyltransferases (Lowe *et al.*, 1990; Goelz *et al.*, 1990). Differential regulation of these fucosyltransferases may explain why on myeloid cells sialyl Lewis X is a marker of differentiation whereas on epithelial cells it is a marker of de-differentiation.

The observation that a ligand for ELAM-1 is expressed on a substantial proportion of carcinomas provokes a possible role for ELAM-1 in hematogenous metastasis. Giavazzi *et al.* (1990) demonstrated a substantial increase in experimental metastases of melanoma cells following pretreatment of mice with IL-1β. This finding, together with previous observations of increased metastases at sites of inflammation in mice (Orr *et al.*, 1985), invokes a role for endothelial cell activation in the promotion of hematogenous metastasis. In support of this view, Taichman and Bevilacqua (manuscript in preparation) have shown that antibodies to the integrin α^4 subunit block an IL-1β-induced increase in the metastasis of B16F10 mouse melanoma cells. One interpretation of these results is that interaction of INCAM-110 on endothelium with $\alpha^4\beta_1$ on the melanoma cells accounts for the IL-1β effect on metastasis. Whether or not cytokine induction of ELAM-1 plays a role in the metastasis of sialyl Lewis X bearing tumor cells remains to be investigated.

VI. Summary

The identification and cloning of ELAM-1 has helped found a new family of vascular adhesion molecules, the SELECTINS, and has provided new insight into the mechanisms of leukocyte–endothelial cell interactions. The importance of ELAM-1 in supporting inflammatory reactions *in vivo* is being investigated in several model systems. The selectivity of the ELAM-1 lectin domain for specific carbohydrate structures on leukocyte surfaces has underscored the growing importance of oligosaccharides in cell–cell adhesion. Further studies of sialyl Lewis X and related carbohydrates present on the surfaces of leukocytes should reveal the mechanisms by which their expression is regulated. The presence of these carbohydrates on some tumor cells is provocative of a role for ELAM-1 in hematogenous metastasis, an issue that is currently being explored. Together, these studies will help to establish the various roles of ELAM-1 in vascular adhesive events.

Acknowledgment

This work was supported by grants from the National Institutes of Health, PO1-HL36028. Dr. Bevilacqua is a PEW Foundation Scholar in the Biomedical Sciences. Dr. Lo is an Irvington House Institute Fellow.

References

Bevilacqua, M. P. (1989). *Circulation* **80(4)**; II–I.
Bevilacqua, M. P., Pober, J. S., Mendrick, D. L., Cotran, R. S., and Gimbrone, M. A. Jr. (1987). *Proc. Natl. Acad. Sci. U.S.A.* 9238–9242.
Bevilacqua, M. P., Stengelin, S., Gimbrone, M. A. Jr., and Seed, B. (1989). *Science* **243**, 1160–1164.
Bonfanti, R., Furie, B. C., Furie, B., and Wagner, D. D. (1989). *Blood* **73**, 1109–1112.
Camerini, D., Jones, S. P., Stamenkovic, I., and Seed, B. (1989). *Nature (London)* **342**, 78–80.
Chandrasekaran, E. V., Davila, M., Nixon, D. W., Goldfarb, M., and Mendicino, J. (1983). *J. Biol. Chem.* **258**, 7213–7222.
Chia, D., Terasaki, P. I., Suyama, N., Galton, J., Hirota, M., and Katz, D. (1985). *Cancer Res.* **45**, 435–437.
Collins, T., Williams, A., Johnston, G. I., Kim, J., Eddy, R., Shows, T., Gimbrone, M. A. Jr., and Bevilacqua, M. P. (1991). *J. Biol. Chem.* **266**, 2466–2473.
Corral, L., Singer, M. S., Macher, B. A., and Rosen, S. D. (1990). *Biochem. Biophys. Res. Commun.* **172**, 1349–1356.
Cotran, R. S., Gimbrone, M. A., Jr., Bevilacqua, M. P., Mendrick, D. L., and Pober, J. S. (1986). *J. Exp. Med.* **164**, 661–666.
Dejana, E., Bertocchi, F., Bortolami, M. C., Regonesi, A., Tonta, A., Breviario, F., and Giavazzi, R. (1988). *J. Clin. Invest.* **82**, 1466–1470.
Drickamer, K. (1988). *J. Biol. Chem.* **263**, 9557–9560.
Elices, M. J., Osborn, L., Takada, Y., Crouse, C., Luhowskyj, S., Helmer, M. E., and Lobb, R. R. (1990). *Cell* **60**, 577–584.
Fukushi, Y., Kannagi, R., Hakomori, S., Shepard, T., Kulander, B. G., and Singer, J. W. (1985). *Cancer Res.* **45**, 3711–3717.
Fukushima, K., Hirota, M., Terasaki, P. I., Wakisaka, A., Togashi, H., Chia, D., Suyama, N., Fukushi, Y., Nudelman, E., and Hakomori, S. (1984). *Cancer Res.* **44**, 5279–5285.
Gallatin, W. M., Weissman, I. L., and Butcher, E. C. (1983). *Nature (London)* **304**, 30–34.
Geng, J. G., Bevilacqua, M. P., Moore, K. L., McIntyre, T. M., Prescott, S. M., Kim, J. M., Bliss, G. A., Zimmerman, G. A., and McEver, R. P. (1990). *Nature (London)* **343**, 757–760.
Giavazzi, R., Garofalo, A., Bani, M. R., Pietro, G., Boraschi, D., Mantovani, A., and Dejana, E. (1990). *Cancer Res.* **50**, 4771–4775.
Goelz, S. E., Hession, C., Goff, D., Griffiths, B., Tizard, R., Newman, B., Chi-Rosso, G., and Lobb, R. (1990). *Cell* **63**, 1136.
Hanisch, F.-G., Uhlenbruck, G., Peter-Katalinic, J., and Egge, H. (1988). *Carbohydrate Res.* **178**, 29–47.
Holmes, E. H., Ostrander, G. K., and Hakomori, S. (1986). *J. Biol. Chem.* **261**, 3737–3743.
Imai, Y., True, D. D., Singer, M. S., and Rosen, S. D. (1990). *J. Cell Biol.* **111**, 1225–1232.
Johnston, I. G., Cook, R. G., and McEver, R. P. (1989). *Cell* **56**, 1033–1044.
Koch, A. E., Burrows, J. C., Haines, G. K., Carlos, T. M., Harlan, J. M., and Leibovich, S. J. (1991). *Lab. Invest.* **64**, 313–320.
Larsen, E., Palabrica, T., Sajer, S., Gilbert, G. E., Wagner, D. D., Furie, B. C., and Furie, B. (1990). *Cell* **63**, 467–474.
Lasky, L. A., Singer, M. S., Yednock, T. A., Dowbenko, D., Fennie, C., Rodriguez, H., Nguyen, T., Stachel, S., and Rosen, S. D. (1989). *Cell* **56**, 1045–1055.
Lewinsohn, D. M., Bargatze, R. F., and Butcher, E. C. (1987). *J. Immunol.* **138**, 4313–4321.
Lowe, J. B., Stoolman, L. M., Nair, R. P., Larse, R. D., Berhend, T. L., and Marks, R. M. (1990). *Cell* **63**, 476–484.
Marlin, S. D., and Springer, T. A. (1987). *Cell* **51**, 813–819.

McEver, R. P., Beckstead, J. H., Moore, K. L., Marshall-Carlson, L., and Bainton, D. F. (1989). *J. Clin. Invest.* **84**, 92–99.
Moore, K. L., Varki, A., and McEver, R. P. (1991). *J. Cell Biol.* **112**, 491–499.
Munro, J. M., Pober, J. S., and Cotran, R. S. (1989). *Am. J. Pathol.* **135**, 121–133.
Munro, J. M., Pober, J. S., and Cotran, R. S. (1991). *Lab. Invest.* **64**, 295–299.
Orr, F. W., Adamson, Y. R., and Young, L. (1985). *Am. Rev. Resp. Dis.* **131**, 607–611.
Osborn, L., Hession, C., Tizard, R., Vassallo, C., Luhowskyj, S., Chi-Rosso, G., and Lobb, R. (1989). *Cell* **59**, 1203–1211.
Phillips, M. L., Nudelman, E., Gaeta, F. C. A., Perez, M., Singhal, A. K., Hakomori, S., and Paulson, J. C. (1990). *Science* **250**, 1130–1132.
Picker, L. J., Kishimoto, T. K., Smith, C. W., Warnock, R. A., and Butcher, E. C. (1991). *Nature (London)* **349**, 796–799.
Pober, J. S., and Cotran, R. S. (1991). *Lab. Invest.* **64**, 301–305.
Rice, G. E., and Bevilacqua, M. P. (1989). *Science* **246**, 1303–1306.
Rice, G. E., Gimbrone, M. A., Jr., Bevilacqua, M. P. (1988). *Am. J. Pathol.* **133**, 204–210
Rice, G. E., Munro, J. M., and Bevilacqua, M. P. (1990). *J. Exp. Med.* **171**, 1369–1374.
Rice, G. E., Munro, J. M., Corless, C., and Bevilacqua, M. P. (1991). *Am. J. Pathol.* **138**, 385–393.
Sharon, N., and Lis, H. (1989). *Science* **246**, 277–234.
Shimizu, Y., Shaw, S., Graber, N., Gopal, T. V., Horgan, K. J., Van Seventer, G. A., and Newman, W. (1991). *Nature (London)* **349**, 799–802.
Siegelman, M., van de Rijn, M., and Weissman, I. L. (1989). *Science* **243**, 1165–1172.
Skubitz, K. M., and Snook, R. W. II. (1987). *J. Immunol.* **139**, 1631–1639.
Smith, C. W., Kishimoto, T. K., Abbass, O., Hughes, B., Rothlein, R., McIntire, L. V., Butcher, E., and Anderson, D. C. (1991). *J. Clin. Invest.* **87**, 609–618.
Staunton, D. E., Dustin, M. L., and Springer, T. A. (1989). *Nature (London)* **359**, 61–64.
Stoolman, L. M. (1989). *Cell* **56**, 907–910.
Symington, F. W., Hedges, D. L., and Hakomori, S. I. (1985). *J. Immunol.* **134**, 2498–2506.
Taichman, D. B., Cybulsky, M. I., Djaffar, I., Longenecker, B. M., Teixido, J., Rice, G. E., Aruffo, A., and Bevilacqua, M. P. (1991). *Cell Regulation* **2**, 347–355.
Tedder, T., Isaacs, C. M., Ernst, T. J., Demetri, G. D., Adler, D. A., and Disteche, C. M. (1989). *J. Exp. Med.* **170**, 123–133.
Tiemeyer, M., Swiedler, S. J., Ishihara, M., Moreland, M., Schweingruber, H., Hirtzer, P., and Brandley, B. K. (1991). *Proc. Natl. Acad. Sci. U.S.A.* **88**, 1138–1142.
Walz, G., Aruffo, A., Kolanus, W., Bevilacqua, M., and Seed, B. (1990). *Science* **250**, 1132–1135.
Watson, M. L., Kingsmore, S. F., Johnston, G. I., Siegelman, M. H., LeBeau, M. M., Lemons, R. S., Bora, N. S., Howard, T. A., Weissman, I. L., McEver, R. P., and Seldin, M. F. (1990). *J. Exp. Med.* **172**, 263–272.

CHAPTER 2

Leukocyte Interactions Mediated by GMP-140

Rodger P. McEver

Department of Medicine
St. Francis Medical Research Institute
University of Oklahoma Health Sciences Center and
Cardiovascular Biology Research Program
Oklahoma Medical Research Foundation
Oklahoma City, Oklahoma 73104

I. Introduction

Endothelial cells, platelets, and leukocytes all play key roles in hemostatic and inflammatory responses to tissue injury. Many of these responses require cellular activation as well as cell–cell contact. This chapter will focus on the properties of GMP-140, a receptor that supports binding of leukocytes to activated platelets and endothelium. GMP-140 mediated adhesive interactions operate in conjunction with cell–cell interactions directed by related molecules and are likely to be important in both hemostatic and inflammatory processes.

II. Tissue and Subcellular Distribution of GMP-140

GMP-140 was originally identified by monoclonal antibodies that reacted only with activated platelets (McEver and Martin, 1984; Hsu-Lin *et al.*,

1984). Immunocytochemistry in conjunction with electron microscopy indicated that the protein was located in membranes of α granules in unstimulated platelets but was redistributed within seconds to the cell surface following activation induced fusion of granule membranes with the plasma membrane (Stenberg *et al.,* 1985; Berman *et al.,* 1986). The protein was named GMP-140 to indicate that it is a granule membrane protein of 140 kd (Stenberg *et al.,* 1985). It has also been referred to as platelet activation dependent granule-external membrane (PADGEM) protein (Berman *et al.,* 1986) and has been given the cluster designation CD62 (Knapp *et al.,* 1989).

Immunoperoxidase analysis of normal human tissues indicated that GMP-140 was present in endothelial cells as well as in platelets and their precursors, megakaryocytes. A striking finding was that the endothelial cell protein was primarily in postcapillary venules, rather than in capillaries or in larger veins, arterioles, or arteries. The protein is synthesized in human umbilical vein endothelial cells, both *in vivo* and *in vitro,* which has facilitated its study (McEver *et al.,* 1989). Endothelial GMP-140 is located in membranes of Weibel–Palade bodies, the secretory granules of endothelium in which large multimers of von Willebrand factor are stored (McEver *et al.,* 1989; Hattori *et al.,* 1989a; Bonfanti *et al.,* 1989). Following cellular activation by agonists such as thrombin or histamine, GMP-140 is rapidly translocated to the cell surface (McEver *et al.,* 1989; Hattori *et al.,* 1989a). Surface appearance is transient, peaking between 3 and 10 minutes, then declining to basal levels over 30 minutes as a result of endocytosis (Hattori *et al.,* 1989a). In contrast, GMP-140 remains on the surface of platelets stimulated *in vitro* for at least 1 hour following stimulation (George *et al.,* 1986); it is not known whether or not endocytosis occurs more rapidly in platelets stimulated *in vivo.*

In summary, GMP-140 is localized in secretory granule membranes of two cell types in the vascular system, platelets and endothelium (Fig. 1). Following activation of these cells by agonists such as thrombin, it is rapidly redistributed to the cell surface. These properties make monoclonal antibodies to GMP-140 useful probes of cellular activation in assays using radioligand binding or flow cytometry (George *et al.,* 1986; Abrams *et al.,* 1990) and potential markers of thrombi *in vivo* with radionuclide imaging procedures (Miller *et al.,* 1991).

III. Structure of GMP-140

GMP-140 is synthesized by cultured endothelial cells and by HEL cells, a human cell line with features of megakaryocytes (McEver *et al.,* 1989;

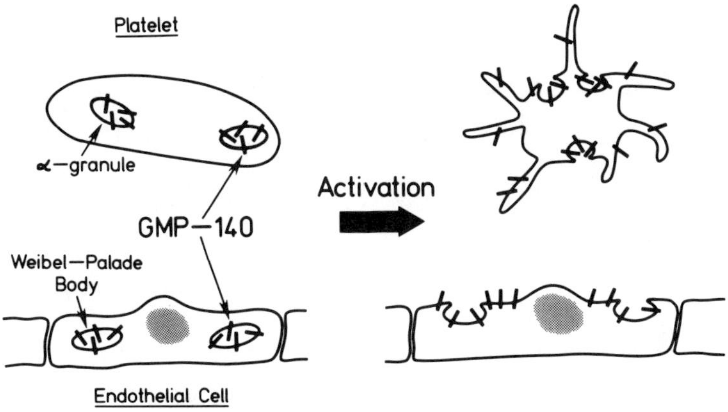

FIGURE 1

Redistribution of GMP-140 following cellular activation. In unstimulated platelets and endothelial cells, GMP-140 is located in membranes of secretory granules: α granules in platelets and Weibel–Palade bodies in endothelial cells. When these cells are stimulated, the granules rapidly fuse with the plasma membrane, release their contents, and express GMP-140 on the cell surface. [Reproduced from McEver (1990) with permission of the publisher.]

Johnston *et al.,* 1989a). Four protein precursors of slightly different apparent Mr are synthesized by metabolically labeled HEL cells (Johnston *et al.,* 1989a). Core high mannose N-linked oligosaccharides are initially added and then processed into larger complex forms. The mature protein contains 30% carbohydrate by weight (Johnston *et al.,* 1989a).

The cDNA-derived amino acid sequence (Johnston *et al.,* 1989b) predicts that GMP-140 is an elongated molecule with a series of cysteine-rich, independently folded domains (Fig. 2). Following a cleavable signal peptide, there is an N-terminal domain homologous to Ca^{2+}-dependent lectins, such as the asialoglycoprotein receptor, then an epidermal growth factor (EGF)-like motif, nine consensus repeats similar to those in complement-regulatory proteins such as CR1, a transmembrane domain, and a short cytoplasmic tail. Nine nucleotide substitutions have been noted in sequences encoding the consensus repeats (Johnston *et al.,* 1989b; Johnston *et al.,* 1990); similar common polymorphisms are present in genes encoding the related repeats of complement regulatory proteins (Hourcade *et al.,* 1989).

The human gene for GMP-140 is located on the long arm of chromosome 1 at bands q21-24 (Watson, *et al.,* 1990). As shown in Fig. 3, the gene

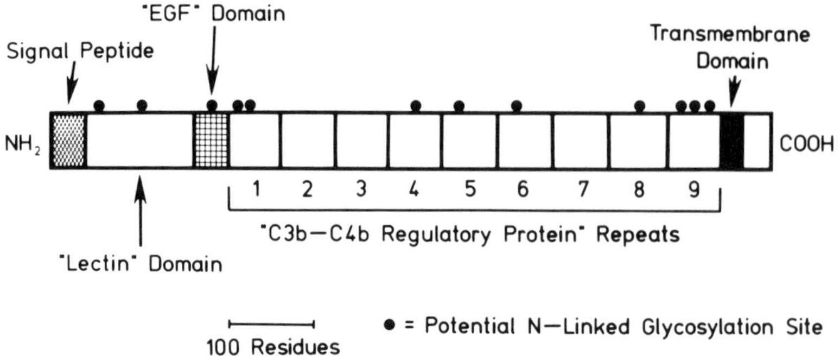

FIGURE 2

Schematic diagram of the domains in GMP-140.
[Reproduced from Johnston *et al.* (1989b) with permission of the publisher.]

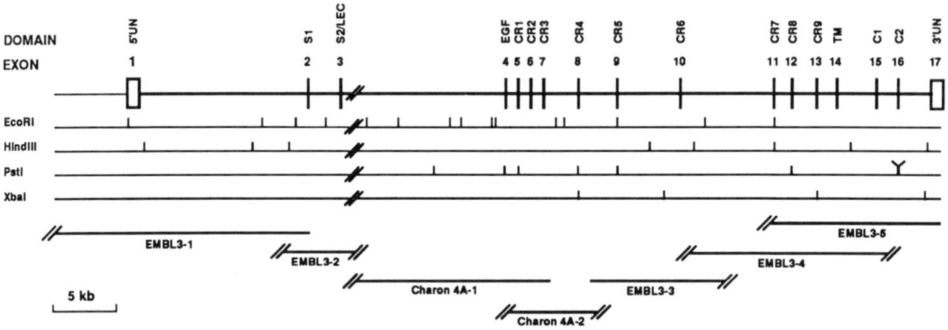

FIGURE 3

Organization of the human gene encoding GMP-140. Exons are indicated by vertical bars, with filled bars representing coding regions and open bars indicating 5'- and 3'-untranslated sequence. The domains encoded by each exon are identified as follows: 5'UN, 5'-untranslated region; S1, first portion of signal peptide; S2/LEC, second portion of signal peptide fused to lectin-like domain; EGF, epidermal growth factor-like domain; CR1 . . . CR9, consensus repeats 1 through 9; TM, transmembrane domain; C1, first portion of cytoplasmic domain; C2, second portion of cytoplasmic domain; 3'UN, 3'-untranslated region. Introns are represented by the thin line and are drawn to scale; the diagonal lines in the intron following exon 3 represent a region of indeterminate length that has not been characterized. A partial restriction map is depicted. At the bottom are shown the positions of seven overlapping genomic clones from which the genomic structure was determined. [Reproduced from Johnston *et al.* (1990) with permission of the publisher.]

spans over 50 kb and contains 17 exons (Johnston *et al.*, 1990). Most exons encode structurally distinct domains, supporting the concept that GMP-140 evolved by exon duplication and rearrangement (Fig. 4). Determination of the genomic structure has helped explain two types of variant cDNA clones previously identified, a rare form with a deletion encoding the seventh consensus repeat and a more common form with a deletion encoding the transmembrane domain (Johnston *et al.*, 1989b). These deletions are precisely encoded by exons, suggesting that the variants arise by alternative splicing of precursor RNA (Fig. 5). The more common variant, which has been found in both platelet and endothelial RNA (Johnston *et al.*, 1990), predicts a soluble form of GMP-140. This potentially important molecule requires further study at the protein level. Very low levels of GMP-140 antigen have been measured in both plasma and serum (K.L. Moore and R.P. McEver, unpublished observations). However, it is not known whether the measured antigen represents proteolytic fragments, GMP-140 associated with vesicles that are not sedimentable in plasma, or the predicted soluble molecule lacking the transmembrane domain.

GMP-140 is structurally related to two vascular cell surface receptors reviewed elsewhere in this volume, endothelial leukocyte adhesion molecule-1 (ELAM-1) (Bevilacqua *et al.*, 1989) and the peripheral lymph node homing receptor (LECAM-1, murine Mel 14 antigen, human Leu 8 antigen, or LAM-1) (Lasky *et al.*, 1989; Siegelman *et al.*, 1989). These three molecules define a new gene family, termed SELECTINS or LECAMs, each of which contains an N-terminal lectin-like domain, followed by an EGF-like domain, consensus repeats (nine in GMP-140, six in ELAM-1, and two in

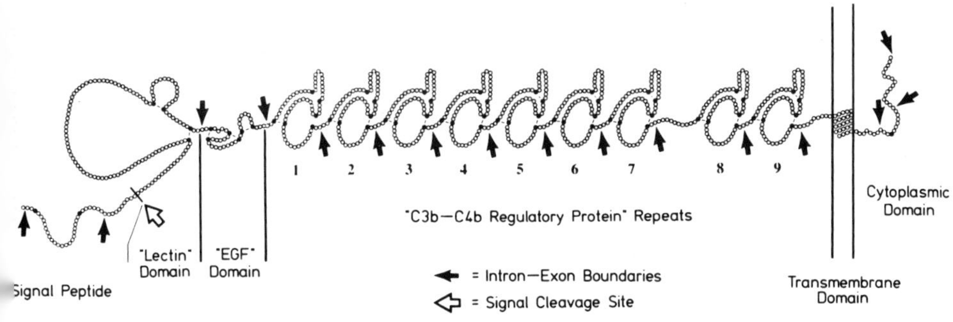

FIGURE 4

Exon–intron boundaries of the gene for GMP-140 shown in relation to the structural domains of the encoded protein. The predicted disulfide bond patterns in each domain are also illustrated. [Reproduced from Johnston *et al.* (1990) with permission of the publisher.]

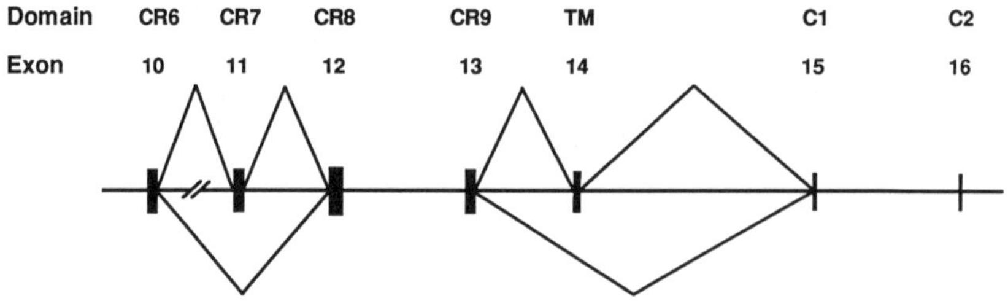

FIGURE 5

Alternative splicing of GMP-140 RNA. The normal splicing pattern producing full-length transcripts is shown above the gene map. Below the gene map are shown alternative splicing events resulting in removal of either exon 11 encoding the seventh consensus repeat or exon 14 encoding the transmembrane domain. Transcripts lacking exon 14 have been detected in both platelets and endothelial cells. The introns are drawn to scale, except for the intron separating exons 10 and 11. [Reproduced from Johnston *et al.* (1990) with permission of the publisher.]

LECAM-1), a transmembrane domain, and a short cytoplasmic tail. The genes have similar intron–exon boundaries, supporting their evolution by gene duplication (Johnston *et al.*, 1990; Ord *et al.*, 1990; Collins *et al.*, 1991). In addition, all three genes are tightly clustered in a 300 kb segment of the equivalent regions of mouse and human chromosome 1, suggesting evolutionary pressure to maintain their proximity (Watson *et al.*, 1990).

IV. Receptor Properties of GMP-140

The SELECTINS all direct interactions of leukocytes with the blood vessel wall during inflammatory responses. The term SELECTINS was proposed because the molecules mediate selective cell–cell contacts by presumed lectin-like mechanisms. LECAM-1 is a leukocyte surface molecule that promotes lymphocyte adhesion to high endothelial venules of peripheral lymph nodes and may support adherence of neutrophils and monocytes to cytokine activated endothelium (See Chapter 3). ELAM-1 is transiently expressed by cytokine activated endothelium where it binds neutrophils and monocytes (See Chapter 1).

Like ELAM-1, GMP-140 is a receptor for neutrophils and monocytes (Fig. 6). Neutrophils bind to purified, immobilized GMP-140 (Geng *et al.*, 1990), to COS cells transfected with GMP-140 cDNA (Geng *et al.*, 1990), and to activated platelets or endothelial cells expressing GMP-140 on their surfaces (Geng *et al.*, 1990; Larsen *et al.*, 1989; Hamburger and McEver, 1990). These interactions are inhibited by monoclonal antibodies to GMP-140 and by fluid-phase GMP-140. Radiolabeled GMP-140 binds reversibly to a saturable number of specific receptors on neutrophils and monocytes, but not on lymphocytes or platelets. Neutrophil activation does not alter receptor number or the apparent affinity of receptors for GMP-140 (Moore *et al.*, 1991).

Several lines of evidence suggest that GMP-140, like the other SELECTINS, actually recognizes oligosaccharide structures on target cells. First, the N-terminal location of the lectin-like domain places it in optimal position for binding to another cell component. Second, fixed or chilled neutrophils bind equally effectively to GMP-140 (Geng *et al.*, 1990; Moore *et al.*, 1991). Third, the epitopes for three monoclonal antibodies to GMP-140 that block neutrophil recognition (Geng *et al.*, 1990) have been mapped to the lectin domain (J.-G. Geng and R.P. McEver, unpublished observations). Fourth, binding of GMP-140 to leukocytes requires Ca^{2+} (Geng *et al.*,

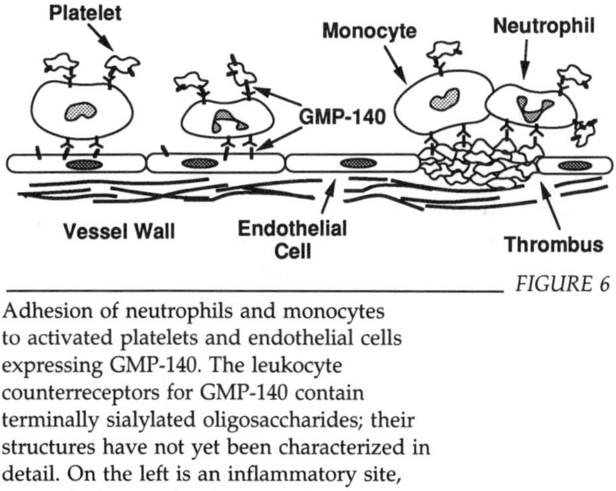

FIGURE 6

Adhesion of neutrophils and monocytes to activated platelets and endothelial cells expressing GMP-140. The leukocyte counterreceptors for GMP-140 contain terminally sialylated oligosaccharides; their structures have not yet been characterized in detail. On the left is an inflammatory site, where leukocytes bind to activated endothelium; the leukocytes, in turn, may recruit activated platelets. On the right is a site of vascular damage and hemorrhage where adherent, activated platelets may bind neutrophils and monocytes. [Reproduced from McEver (1991) with permission of the publisher.]

1990; Larsen *et al.*, 1989; Hamburger and McEver, 1990; Moore *et al.*, 1991), a finding consistent with the Ca^{2+}-dependent carbohydrate recognition of known lectins with similar structures (Drickamer, 1988).

If GMP-140 is a lectin, it could potentially bind to glycoproteins, glycolipids on the plasma membranes of leukocytes, or both. However, pretreatment of neutrophils with proteases completely inhibits binding of [^{125}I]GMP-140 (Moore *et al.*, 1991), suggesting that the relevant recognition structures are carried by proteins rather than lipids on these cells. Binding is inhibited by high concentrations of mannose-1-phosphate and certain anionic polysaccharides (Moore *et al.*, 1991; Skinner *et al.*, 1990), providing supporting but not unequivocal evidence for a lectin-like interaction.

More direct evidence for interaction of GMP-140 with carbohydrates comes from the observation that pretreatment of neutrophils with neuraminidases reduces binding of radiolabeled GMP-140 (Moore *et al.*, 1991). This suggests that sialic acid constitutes an essential feature of the receptor for GMP-140. Binding is reduced by neuraminidase from Vibrio cholera, which cleaves sialic acid at α2,3, α2,6, and α2,8 linkages, and from Newcastle disease virus, which cleaves only α2,3 and α2,8 linkages (Moore *et al.*, 1991). Since neutrophils do not contain α2,8 linkages, at least some of the sialic residues appear to be linked α2,3 in the structure recognized by GMP-140. Broad-spectrum neuraminidases also prevent rosetting of activated platelets with neutrophils, a GMP-140 mediated adhesive event. However, neuraminidase from Newcastle disease virus did not prevent rosetting (Corral *et al.*, 1990). Because the latter enzyme is associated with an intact virus which itself binds to cells, it may have directly agglutinated platelets with neutrophils even though it removed a sialic acid linkage required for GMP-140 binding.

It has been reported that the oligosaccharide receptor for GMP-140 is the abundant myeloid structure Lewis x (Le^x) (CD15, lacto-N-fucopentaose III) (Larsen *et al.*, 1990). The core component of this structure, Galβ1,4[Fucα1, 3]GlcNAcβ1,3-, is found on glycolipids and several different glycoproteins on neutrophils, generally as part of repeating units in polylactosamine chains (Fukuda, 1985). The evidence for recognition of Le^x by GMP-140 was based on the observation that antiCD15 antibodies or high concentrations of LNFIII inhibited adhesion of myeloid cells to activated platelets or to GMP-140 transfected cells. Since the neuraminidase studies implicate sialic acid residues in recognition (Moore *et al.*, 1991; Corral *et al.*, 1990), it is clear that Le^x per se cannot be the receptor for GMP-140. Furthermore, the protease studies suggest that the critical structure is carried on proteins rather than lipids, whereas Le^x is found on both glycolipids and glycoproteins. Finally, binding of radiolabeled GMP-140 to neutrophils is not inhibited by antibodies to CD15 or by a multivalent glycoconjugate consisting of Le^x coupled to albumin by a spacer (Moore *et al.*, 1991). Therefore, while the Le^x structure might constitute part of the oligosaccharide receptor for GMP-140, it alone cannot provide the required affinity and specificity.

The carbohydrate receptor for the related selectin, ELAM-1, has been reported to be sialyl Le^x, which contains a sialic acid linked $\alpha 2,3$ to the Le^x structure (Phillips *et al.*, 1990; Walz *et al.*, 1990; Lowe *et al.*, 1990; Tiemeyer *et al.*, 1990). This terminal oligosaccharide is also a candidate receptor for GMP-140. However, a sialyl Le^x glycoconjugate does not inhibit binding of radiolabeled GMP-140 to neutrophils (Moore *et al.*, 1991) and antibodies to sialyl Le^x do not inhibit rosetting of activated platelets with neutrophils (Corral *et al.*, 1990). Therefore, detailed characterization of the oligosaccharide receptor for GMP-140 requires further study. It is an attractive hypothesis that all three SELECTINS bind sialylated fucosylated structures. These structures may be related but are unlikely to be identical. Binding interactions mediated by GMP-140 and LECAM-1, respectively, show some differences in their ability to be inhibited by specific charged monosaccharides and polysaccharides (Moore *et al.*, 1991). Furthermore, fluid-phase GMP-140 inhibits neutrophil adhesion to activated endothelial cells expressing GMP-140 but not to cells expressing ELAM-1 (Gamble *et al.*, 1990; Zimmerman *et al.*, 1990b).

GMP-140 requires at least two Ca^{2+}-binding sites for optimal interaction with leukocytes (Geng *et al.*, 1990). It is possible that Ca^{2+} binds to both the lectin and EGF domains of GMP-140, since both types of motifs have been shown to bind Ca^{2+} in other proteins (Loeb and Drickamer, 1988; Persson *et al.*, 1989). Perhaps the affinity and specificity of the interaction of GMP-140 with its receptor is due to protein–carbohydrate binding mediated by the lectin domain and protein–protein binding mediated by the EGF domain. Alternatively, the EGF domain may modulate the conformation of the lectin domain to produce a Ca^{2+}-dependent, highly specific interaction with an oligosaccharide receptor. In this model, the consensus repeats may mediate other functions not yet characterized. They may also position the lectin domain at a sufficient distance from the platelet or endothelial membrane to allow efficient binding to its receptor on leukocytes.

V. Physiologic Role of GMP-140

During inflammation, leukocytes must first adhere to endothelium, then migrate into tissues at sites of infection or injury. This is a temporally regulated process, with migration of neutrophils and monocytes occurring earlier than lymphocytes. Because GMP-140 is constitutively synthesized by endothelium and stored in Weibel–Palade bodies, it can be translocated to the cell surface within minutes after endothelial stimulation with agonists such as thrombin or histamine. Therefore, it is likely to be the first leukocyte adhesion molecule expressed by activated endothelium during acute inflammation. The surface exposure of GMP-140 is also transient because of endocytosis of the receptor within 30 minutes after its initial appearance. This leads to rapid dampening of the proinflammatory surface on the endothelium. Persistent infection or tissue injury leads to the elaboration of inflammatory cytokines that induce synthesis and surface expression of ELAM-1 during the next 4 to 6 hours (Bevilacqua *et al.*, 1987). GMP-140 and ELAM-1 may, therefore, work in concert to direct early, regionally specific adherence of neutrophils and monocytes at sites of acute inflammation.

Migration of neutrophils into injured tissues requires the leukocyte β2 integrins or CD11/CD18 molecules, as dramatically illustrated in patients with leukocyte adhesion deficiency. These patients, who are congenitally deficient in the β2 integrins, fail to accumulate neutrophils at inflammatory sites and, therefore, suffer frequent severe infections (Anderson and Springer, 1987). Although they are constitutively present on the plasma membrane, the CD11/CD18 molecules require neutrophil activation before they can bind to counterreceptors on the endothelial cell surface (Lo *et al.*, 1989).

The phospholipid signaling molecule, platelet activating factor (PAF), is a potent neutrophil agonist. PAF is rapidly synthesized and delivered to the cell surface when the endothelium is activated by thrombin or histamine. The expression of PAF is transient because of rapid degradation by a plasma PAF specific hydrolase (Prescott *et al.*, 1990). Because the kinetics of surface expression of PAF and GMP-140 are so similar, it appeared likely that the two molecules could cooperate to promote neutrophil adhesion and migration. This hypothesis is supported by several observations. Neutrophil adhesion to thrombin activated endothelium is partially inhibited by antibodies to CD18 (Zimmerman and McIntyre, 1988). Although adhesion of neutrophils to GMP-140 does not require CD11/CD18 molecules, adherence of PAF stimulated neutrophils to endothelium is absolutely dependent on these integrins (Zimmerman *et al.*, 1990b). Antibodies to GMP-140 and competitive PAF receptor antagonists each partially block neutrophil adhesion to thrombin or histamine stimulated endothelium, whereas combining both inhibitors completely prevents adhesion (Zimmerman *et al.*, 1990a; Zimmerman *et al.*, 1990b). These observations suggest that GMP-140 expressed by rapidly activated endothelium promotes attachment of circulating unstimulated neutrophils, which are then positioned for activation by PAF. The activated neutrophils develop competent CD11/CD18 molecules that bind to endothelial cell counterreceptors, facilitating spreading and migration of the cells into underlying tissues.

The two-step model of neutrophil adhesion followed by activation assumes that binding of GMP-140 does not prevent subsequent neutrophil activation by PAF. It has been proposed that GMP-140 acts as a natural anti-inflammatory agent, based on observations that the fluid phase protein prevents adhesion of neutrophils activated by tumor necrosis factor (Gamble *et al.*, 1990). However, fluid phase GMP-140 clearly does not inhibit adhesion to endothelium of neutrophils stimulated by PAF or the bacterial chemotactic peptide fMLP, indicating that GMP-140 does not globally prevent neutrophil activation (Zimmerman *et al.*, 1990b).

Unlike the other SELECTINS, GMP-140 is also expressed on the surface of activated platelets, where it mediates binding of these cells to neutrophils and monocytes (Larsen *et al.*, 1989; Hamburger and McEver, 1990). The physiologic significance of this process is not established, but there are several possibilities. *In vivo,* neutrophils support emigration of platelets into acute inflammatory sites (Issekutz *et al.*, 1983); this phenomenon might require GMP-140 mediated contacts between neutrophils and activated platelets. The recruitment of platelets could be useful, because these cells release inflammatory mediators such as platelet factor 4 and platelet derived growth factor (Weksler, 1988). At sites of vessel injury, neutrophils and monocytes have been observed adhering to platelet aggregates, an interaction potentially dependent on GMP-140 (Henry, 1961). Activated monocytes may promote thrombin generation by developing a surface for prothrombinase components and by expressing tissue factor, the key initiator of the extrinsic pathway of coagulation (Edwards and Rickles, 1984). Close contact between platelets and neutrophils may facilitate transcellular metabolism of leukotrienes and lipoxins that are not produced by either cell type alone (Maclouf and Murphy, 1988; Serhan and Sheppard, 1990; Marcus, 1990). Finally, expression of GMP-140 may provide a mechanism for rapid clearance of activated platelets from the circulation by macrophages in the reticuloendothelial system.

VI. Pathologic Role of GMP-140

Excessive accumulation of neutrophils has been implicated in a number of inflammatory disorders, including acute respiratory distress syndrome, ischemia-reperfusion injury, gram-negative septic shock, and rheumatoid arthritis (Malech and Gallin, 1987). Tissue injury is thought to result from release of oxygen free radicals and proteases from activated neutrophils (Mullane *et al.,* 1988; Henson and Johnston, 1987). The endothelium is likely to be particularly susceptible to damage because of certain unique biochemical features and its proximity to circulating neutrophils (Ward and Varani, 1990). Neutrophils adherent to some surfaces release much larger quantities of free radicals in response to agonists than they do when in suspension (Nathan *et al.,* 1989). In physiologic inflammation, leukocytes adhere only transiently to endothelium before migrating into tissues, thus lessening the risk of vascular damage. Unregulated expression of adhesion molecules, however, might lead to persistent adherence and activation of neutrophils. If so, interruption of leukocyte adhesion mechanisms may reduce tissue injury, whatever the proximal cause of disease.

Pathologic inflammatory sites, for example, ischemic regions due to ruptured atherosclerotic plaque, may produce mediators such as thrombin that can activate platelets and endothelial cells and expose GMP-140. Nonphysiologic mediators may also be released that can activate these cells. Insertion of the terminal complement components C5b-9 into cellular membranes activates both platelets and endothelial cells, leading to granule secretion, expression of GMP-140, and release of procoagulant microvesicles (Hattori *et al.,* 1989b). Low concentrations of oxygen radicals induce prolonged exposure of GMP-140 on the endothelial cell surface, leading to enhanced neutrophil adherence over several hours (Patel *et al.,* 1991). *In vivo,* this unregulated expression of GMP-140 could result in sustained neutrophil recruitment, additional production of oxygen radicals by adherent cells, and eventual tissue destruction.

Some malignant cells may metastasize by using adhesion mechanisms normally used for leukocyte recruitment. Based on indirect evidence, lectin–carbohydrate interactions have been proposed to promote spreading of certain experimental tumors (Lotan and Raz, 1988). In another study, a human colon carcinoma cell line has been shown to bind specifically to ELAM-1 (Rice and Bevilacqua, 1989). Other malignant cells may potentially express receptors for GMP-140. Malignant cell-surface display of receptors for leukocyte adhesion molecules may target spread of tumors to endothelium at inflammatory sites, where expression of adhesion molecules such as GMP-140 and ELAM-1 might be induced. Platelets have also been shown to promote experimental tumor metastasis (Boukerche *et al.,* 1989). Although the molecules described to date are integrins, there may be examples where platelet adhesion to tumor cells is mediated by GMP-140.

Appropriate *in vivo* models of inflammation, metastasis, and thrombosis are required to evaluate the participation of GMP-140 and other adhesion molecules in disease. Should their pathologic roles be confirmed, new drugs might be designed to interrupt their function. Such pharmaceuticals might include monoclonal antibodies, peptides, oligosaccharides, or recombinant soluble proteins, variously designed to block adhesion molecules on endothelium, leukocytes, platelets, or tumor cells.

Acknowledgment

Supported by grant HL 34364 and a Research Career Development Award from the National Institutes of Health.

References

Abrams, C. S., Ellison, N., Budzynski, A. Z., and Shattil, S. J. (1990). *Blood* **75,** 128–138.

Anderson, D. C., and Springer, T. A. (1987). *Ann. Rev. Med.* **38,** 175–194.

Berman, C. L., Yeo, E. L., Wencel-Drake, J. D., Furie, B. C., Ginsberg, M. H., and Furie, B. (1986). *J. Clin. Invest.* **78,** 130–137.

Bevilacqua, M. P., Pober, J. S., Mendrick, D. L., Cotran, R. S., and Gimbrone, M. A., Jr. (1987). *Proc. Natl. Acad. Sci. U.S.A.* **84,** 9238–9242.

Bevilacqua, M. P., Stengelin, S., Gimbrone, M. A., Jr., and Seed, B. (1989). *Science* **243,** 1160–1165.

Bonfanti, R., Furie, B. C., Furie, B., and Wagner, D. D. (1989). *Blood* **73,** 1109–1112.

Boukerche, H., Berthier-Vergnes, O., Tabone, E., Dore, J.-F., Leung, L. L. K., and McGregor, J. L. (1989). *Blood* **74,** 658–663.

Collins, T., Williams, A., Johnston, G. I., Kim, J., Eddy, R., Shows, T., Gimbrone, M. A., Jr., and Bevilacqua, M. P. (1991). *J. Biol. Chem.* **266,** 2466–2473.

Corral, L., Singer, M. S., Macher, B. A., and Rosen, S. D. (1990). *Biochem. Biophys. Res. Commun.* **172,** 1349–1356.

Drickamer, K. (1988). *J. Biol. Chem.* **263,** 9557–9560.

Edwards, R. L., and Rickles, F. R. (1984). *In* "Progress in Hemostasis and Thrombosis" (T. H. Spaet, ed.), 2nd ed., pp. 183–209. Grune and Stratton, New York.

Fukuda, M. (1985). *Biochem. Biophys. Acta* **780,** 119–150.

Gamble, J. R., Skinner, M. P., Berndt, M. C., and Vadas, M. A. (1990). *Science* **249,** 414–417.

Geng, J.-G., Bevilacqua, M. P., Moore, K. L., McIntyre, T. M., Prescott, S. M., Kim, J. M., Bliss, G. A., Zimmerman, G. A., and McEver, R. P. (1990). *Nature* **343,** 757–760.

George, J. N., Pickett, E. B., Saucerman, S., McEver, R. P., Kunicki, T. J., Kieffer, N., and Newman, P. J. (1986). *J. Clin. Invest.* **78,** 340–348.

Hamburger, S. A., and McEver, R. P. (1990). *Blood* **75,** 550–554.

Hattori, R., Hamilton, K. K., Fugate, R. D., McEver, R. P., and Sims, P. J. (1989a). *J. Biol. Chem.* **264,** 7768–7771.

Hattori, R., Hamilton, K. K., McEver, R. P., and Sims, P. J. (1989b). *J. Biol. Chem.* **264,** 9053–9060.

Henry, R. L. (1961). *Thromb. Diath. Haemorrh.* **13,** 35–46.

Henson, P. M., and Johnston, R. B., Jr. (1987). *J. Clin. Invest.* **79,** 669–674.
Hourcade, D., Holers, V. M., and Atkinson, J. P. (1989). *In* "Advances in Immunology," Vol. 45 (F. J. Dixon, ed.), pp. 381–416. Academic Press, New York.
Hsu-Lin, S.-C., Berman, C. L., Furie, B. C., August, D., and Furie, B. (1984). *J. Biol. Chem.* **259,** 9121–9126.
Issekutz, A. C., Ripley, M., and Jackson, J. R. (1983). *Lab. Invest.* **49,** 716–724.
Johnston, G. I., Kurosky, A., and McEver, R. P. (1989a). *J. Biol. Chem.* **264,** 1816–1823.
Johnston, G. I., Cook, R. G., and McEver, R. P. (1989b). *Cell* **56,** 1033–1044.
Johnston, G. I., Bliss, G. A., Newman, P. J., and McEver, R. P. (1990). *J. Biol. Chem.* **265,** 21381–21385.
Knapp, W., Dorken, B., Rieber, P., Schmidt, R. E., Stein, H., and von dem Borne, A. E. G. Kr. (1989). *Blood* **74,** 1448–1450.
Larsen, E., Celi, A., Gilbert, G. E., Furie, B. C., Erban, J. K., Bonfanti, R., Wagner, D. D., and Furie, B. (1989). *Cell* **59,** 305–312.
Larsen, E., Palabrica, T., Sajer, S., Gilbert, G. E., Wagner, D. D., Furie, B. C., and Furie, B. (1990). *Cell* **63,** 467–474.
Lasky, L. A., Singer, M. S., Yednock, T. A., Dowbenko, D., Fennie, C., Rodriguez, H., Nguyen, T., Stachel, S., and Rosen, S. D. (1989). *Cell* **56,** 1045–1055.
Lo, S. K., Van Seventer, G. A., Levin, S. M., and Wright, S. D. (1989). *J. Immunol.* **143,** 3325–3329.
Loeb, J. A., and Drickamer, K. (1988). *J. Biol. Chem.* **263,** 9752–9760.
Lotan, R., and Raz, A. (1988). *J. Cell. Biochem.* **37,** 107–117.
Lowe, J. B., Stoolman, L. M., Nair, R. P., Larsen, R. D., Berhend, T. L., and Marks, R. M. (1990). *Cell* **63,** 475–484.
McEver, R. P. (1990). *Blood Cells* **16,** 73–83.
McEver, R. P. (1991). *J. Cell Biochem.* **45,** 156–161.
McEver, R. P., Beckstead, J. H., Moore, K. L., Marshall-Carlson, L., and Bainton, D. F. (1989). *J. Clin. Invest.* **84,** 92–99.
McEver, R. P., and Martin, M. N. (1984). *J. Biol. Chem.* **259,** 9799–9804.
Maclouf, J. A., and Murphy, R. C. (1988). *J. Biol. Chem.* **263,** 174–181.
Malech, H. L., and Gallin, J. I. (1987). *N. Engl. J. Med.* **317,** 687–694.
Marcus, A. J. (1990). *Methods Enzymol.* **187,** 585–598.
Miller, D. D., Boulet, A. J., Tio, F. O., Garcia, O. J., McEver, R. P., Palmaz, J. C., Pak, K. Y., Neblock, D. S., Berger, H. J., and Daddona, P. E. (1991). *Circulation* **83,** 224–236.
Moore, K. L., Varki, A., and McEver, R. P. (1991). *J. Cell Biol.* **112,** 491–499.
Mullane, K. M., Westlin, W., and Kraemer, R. (1988). *Ann. N. Y. Acad. Sci.* **524,** 103–121.
Nathan, C., Srimal, S., Farber, C., Sanchez, E., Kabbash, L., Asch, A., Gailit, J., and Wright, S. D. (1989). *J. Cell Biol.* **109,** 1341–1349.
Ord, D. C., Ernst, T. J., Zhou, L.-J., Rambaldi, A., Spertini, O., Griffin, J., and Tedder, T. F. (1990). *J. Biol. Chem.* **265,** 7760–7767.
Patel, K. D., Zimmerman, G. A., Prescott, S. M., McEver, R. P., and McIntyre, T. M. (1991). *J. Cell Biol.* **112,** 749–759.
Persson, E., Selander, M., Linse, S., Drakenberg, T., Ohlin, A.-K., and Stenflo, J. (1989). *J. Biol. Chem.* **264,** 16897–16904.
Phillips, M. L., Nudelman, E., Gaeta, F. C. A., Perez, M., Singhal, A. K., Hakomori, S., and Paulson, J. C. (1990). *Science* **250,** 1130–1132.
Prescott, S. M., Zimmerman, G. A., and McIntyre, T. M. (1990). *J. Biol. Chem.* **265,** 17381–17384.
Rice, G. E., and Bevilacqua, M. P. (1989). *Science* **246,** 1303–1306.
Serhan, C. N. and Sheppard, K.-A. (1990). *J. Clin. Invest.* **85,** 772–780.
Siegelman, M. H., van de Rijn, M., and Weissman, I. L. (1989). *Science* **243,** 1165–1172.

Skinner, M. P., Lucas, C. M., Burns, G. F., Chesterman, C. N., and Berndt, M. C. (1990). *Circulation* **82,** III–598. (Abstract).

Stenberg, P. E., McEver, R. P., Shuman, M. A., Jacques, Y. V., and Bainton, D. F. (1985). *J. Cell Biol.* **101,** 880–886.

Tiemeyer, M., Swiedler, S. J., Ishihara, M., Moreland, M., Schweingruber, H., Hirtzer, P., and Brandley, B. K. (1991). *Proc. Natl. Acad. Sci. U.S.A.* **88,** 1138–1142.

Walz, G., Aruffo, A., Kolanus, W., Bevilacqua, B., and Seed, B. (1990). *Science* **250,** 1132–1135.

Ward, P. A. and Varani, J. (1990). *J. Leukocyte Biol.* **48,** 97–102.

Watson, M. L., Kingsmore, S. F., Johnston, G. I., Siegelman, M. H., Le Beau, M. M., Lemons, R. S., Bora, N. S., Howard, T. A., Weissman, I. L., McEver, R. P., and Seldin, M. F. (1990). *J. Exp. Med.* **172,** 263–272.

Weksler, B. B. (1988). *In* "Platelet Membrane Receptors: Molecular Biology, Biochemistry, and Pathology" (G. A. Jamieson, ed.), pp. 611–638. Alan R. Liss, Inc., New York.

Zimmerman, G. A., and McIntyre, T. M. (1988). *J. Clin. Invest.* **81,** 531–537.

Zimmerman, G. A., McIntyre, T. M., Mehra, M., and Prescott, S. M. (1990a). *J. Cell Biol.* **110,** 529–540.

Zimmerman, G. A., McIntyre, T. M., Prescott, S. M., McEver, R. P., and Patel, K. D. (1990b). *Proc. First Internatl. Cong. Inflam.* (Abstract).

CHAPTER 3

Leukocyte Adhesion Molecule-1 (LAM-1): Structure, Function, Genetics, and Evolution

Geoffrey S. Kansas, Olivier Spertini, and Thomas F. Tedder

Division of Tumor Immunology
Dana-Farber Cancer Institute and
Department of Pathology
Harvard Medical School
Boston, Massachusetts 02115

I. Introduction

Mature T and B lymphocytes continually travel between the secondary lymphoid organs and the blood, a process termed lymphocyte recirculation. The first step in leaving the blood and entering a lymph node or other lymphoid organ is the binding of the lymphocyte to the luminal surface of specialized, high-walled endothelial cells in the postcapillary venules of most secondary lymphoid organs. These venules are termed high endothelial venules (HEV) and the lymphocyte molecules that mediate this initial binding are termed homing receptors. An important advance in the study of lymphocyte recirculation was the ability to study the initial binding of lymphocytes to HEV using an *in vitro* assay developed by Stamper and Woodruff (1976). In this assay, lymphocytes are overlaid onto frozen histological sections of lymph node or other tissue, the sections are incubated under rotation at low temperatures, fixed, gently washed, and the lymphocytes adhering to the HEV are quantitated. The use of this assay system has been critical in demonstrating the existence of at least two organ specific pathways of lymphocyte adhesion to HEV, one involving peripheral lymph nodes and other "nonmucosal" organs, and one involving Peyer's patch and other mucosal sites (Berg *et al.*, 1989; Stoolman, 1990; Chin *et al.*, 1984; Yednock and Rosen, 1989).

The Stamper–Woodruff assay was also crucial in identifying the leukocyte and endothelial cell surface molecules that participate in lymphocyte adhesion to HEV. The molecules that function as HEV receptors can be included among an increasing number of leukocyte adhesion molecules that act in a coordinated manner to orchestrate the migration of various classes of leukocytes during lymphocyte recirculation, inflammation, metastasis, and other types of leukocyte traffic. These receptors include representatives of at least three gene families or superfamilies (Hemler, 1988; Springer, 1990): The integrins, the immunoglobulin superfamily, and the SELECTIN/LEC-CAM family. This review will focus primarily on leukocyte adhesion molecule-1 (LAM-1) (Tedder *et al.*, 1989), a member of the SELECTIN family that is the human counterpart of the murine peripheral lymph node homing receptor identified by the MEL-14 antibody (Gallatin *et al.*, 1983) and the role of LAM-1 in the regulation of leukocyte traffic in man. Many comprehensive reviews are available describing the expression and function of the MEL-14 antigen, so much of that work, which laid the foundation for studies on LAM-1, will not be reviewed in this report.

II. LAM-1 Structure

LAM-1 was first identified structurally by cDNA cloning (Tedder *et al.*, 1989; Bowen *et al.*, 1989; Siegelman and Weissman, 1989) that revealed a protein composed of an interesting and unique mosaic of domain motifs (Fig. 1). This includes an aminoterminal C-type lectin domain, followed by an epidermal growth factor (EGF)-like domain, two short consensus repeat units (SCR) homologous to those found in C3/C4 binding proteins, a potential transmembrane region, and a cytoplasmic tail. The structure of this protein immediately suggested a role for this putative cell–surface molecule in cell–cell interactions, and this new molecule was, therefore, named the leukocyte adhesion molecule-1. Although human lymphocytes were known to express a receptor functionally homologous with the mur-

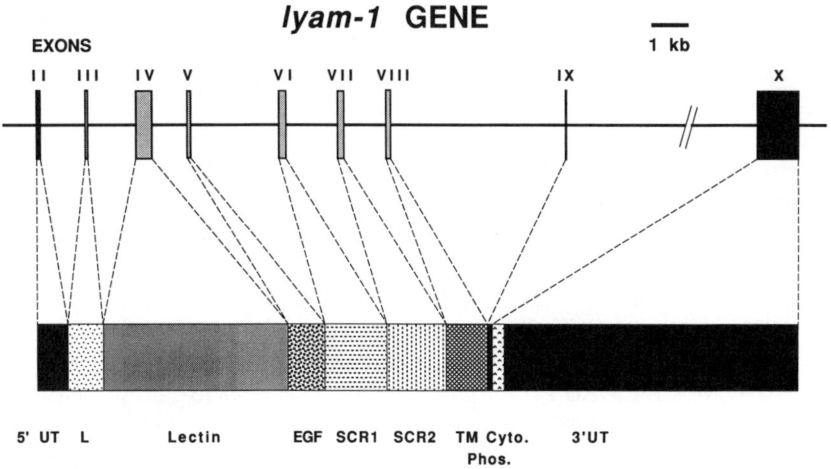

FIGURE 1

Structure of the *lyam-1* gene and LAM-1 cDNAs. The exons (II through IX) that encode LAM-1 domains are shown: 5′ UT, 5′ untranslated region; L, leader peptide; EGF, EGF-like domain; TM, transmembrane; Phos., the potential phosphorylation cassette; Cyto., cytoplasmic domain; 3′ UT, the 3′ untranslated region of the cDNAs.

ine MEL-14 antigen, the human counterpart had previously been suggested to be the CD44 cell–surface antigen (Jalkanen *et al.,* 1986; Jalkanen *et al.,* 1987). However, CD44 was shown to be the hyaluronic acid receptor (Miyake *et al.,* 1990), and the cDNA sequence of CD44 is unrelated to LAM-1, MEL-14, or to the other SELECTINS (Goldstein *et al.,* 1989; Stamenkovic *et al.,* 1989).

A. Structure of LAM-1 and Other SELECTINS

The lectin-like domain of LAM-1 is homologous with other carbohydrate binding proteins, including asialoglycoprotein receptors and mannose binding proteins, and this domain contains essentially all of the invariant residues found in C-type animal lectin carbohydrate recognition domains (Drickamer, 1988). Consistent with this, Stoolman, Rosen and colleagues have demonstrated that both murine and human homing receptors required Ca^{++} to function (Stoolman and Ebling, 1989; Stoolman *et al.,* 1987). In contrast to LAM-1, most C-type lectin domains are contained within type II membrane proteins and are thus found at the carboxy terminal end of the molecule. The EGF-like domain contains the 6 Cys residues conserved in all EGF-like repeats and is 39% identical in amino acid sequence to EGF. Because EGF-like domains are found in several proteins, where they mediate protein–protein interactions, it is possible that the EGF domain of LAM-1 is involved in ligand binding and is not merely a structural feature of this molecule. The SCR of LAM-1 and the other SELECTINS are unique in that, in contrast to all other previously described SCR, they contain an additional pair of conserved Cys residues. It is likely that this feature plays an important structural role, as previous work has demonstrated the rodlike nature of many proteins containing SCR domains (e.g., CD35). Additionally, it is possible that these tandem SCR function in binding interactions, because the minimum protein binding unit in the C3/C4 binding proteins are composed of two tandem SCR. Thus, LAM-1 truly represents a structurally unique protein.

LAM-1 and the MEL-14 antigen are 77% identical in amino acid sequence (Tedder *et al.*, 1989; Laskey *et al.*, 1989; Siegelman *et al.*, 1989). The two SCRs of the MEL-14 antigen are identical in amino acid sequence while those of LAM-1 are 61% identical. A domain organization similar to that of LAM-1/MEL-14 is also found in two other leukocyte adhesion proteins in man: ELAM-1, which is expressed by activated endothelium and mediates the binding of these cells to myeloid cells (Bevilacqua *et al.*, 1989); and CD62 (PADGEM, GMP-140), which is found on activated platelets and endothelium, and mediates the binding of these cells to monocytes and neutrophils (Johnston *et al.*, 1989; Larsen *et al.*, 1990). This group of proteins has been termed the SELECTIN or LEC-CAM family. Remarkably, reports from multiple groups describing the cloning of cDNAs for LAM-1, the MEL-14 antigen, CD62, and ELAM-1 were all submitted for publication essentially simultaneously (Tedder *et al.*, 1989; Bowen *et al.*, 1989; Laskey *et al.*, 1989; Bevilacquas *et al.*, 1989; Johnston *et al.*, 1989). The principal structural difference between these three adhesion proteins is the number of SCR: ELAM-1 has six, and CD62 has nine. Amino acid sequences of the lectin domains of CD62 and ELAM-1 are 67 and 61% identical with LAM-1 and also show lower levels (30 to 40%) of homology to other C-type animal lectin domains. For comparison, the lectin domain of LAM-1 shows 83% sequence identity with that of the murine homologue, MEL-14. The EGF-like domains of the SELECTINS exhibit 61 to 64% homology, and the SCR show a lower level of homology (~35 to 45%).

A striking feature is that the region of greatest homology between LAM-1 and the MEL-14 antigen is in the region consisting of the transmembrane domain and the cytoplasmic tail, which collectively are 88% homologous. These regions in ELAM-1 and CD62 are not homologous with LAM-1. Although no direct data exist, the fact that LAM-1 and MEL-14 are the only SELECTINs shed from the cell surface following cellular activation (indeed, ELAM-1 and PADGEM are only expressed at the cell surface following activation) makes it likely that this region is of critical importance in this phenomenon and also in the regulation of LAM-1 function.

B. Structure of the Gene That Encodes LAM-1

The structure of the *lyam-1* gene was determined by isolating overlapping genomic DNA clones that hybridized with LAM-1 cDNAs (Ord *et al.*, 1990). Although the complete size of the *lyam-1* gene is unknown, restriction map analysis and nucleotide sequencing of the cloned DNAs revealed that the *lyam-1* gene spans greater than 30 kb of DNA and encodes at least 10 exons. Exons II through X encode translated sequences as follows: Exon II encodes the translation initiation codon; exon III, the leader peptide; exon IV, the lectin domain; exon V, the EGF-like domain; exons VI and VII, the SCRs; exon VIII, the transmembrane region; exon IX, a portion of the cytoplasmic tail that may serve as a site for phosphorylation; and exon X, the terminus of the cytoplasmic tail and the 3′ untranslated region of the mRNA (Fig. 1). Therefore, the *lyam-1* gene is assembled from individual exons encoding distinct structural or functional units. Thus, the genomic structure of the LAM-1 gene is a clear example of a case where introns have facilitated the shuffling of distinct exons from several ancestral proteins to form a unique protein of unrelated overall structure and function. The lectin, EGF and SCR domains of ELAM-1 and CD62 show an identical exon/intron organization as described for LAM-1 (Collins *et al.*, 1991; Johnston *et al.*, 1990).

The *lyam-1* gene is located on chromosome 1 at band q23-25 (Tedder *et al.*, 1989). This region is distinct from the "complement receptor" locus at band 1q32 that encodes the SCR containing protein, CD35 (CR1), CD21 (CR2), C4-binding protein, and factor H. The genes for the other SELECTINs, ELAM-1 and CD62, are also located within this region (Johnston *et al.*, 1990; Collins *et al.*, 1991) and are arranged in tandem along chromosome 1 with *lyam-1* (Watson *et al.*, 1990). Thus, it is likely that this family of adhesion receptors evolved from a common precursor through gene duplication and exon amplification.

A novel and unique cDNA encoding a putative PI-linked form of LAM-1 has been described by others (Camerini *et al.*, 1989). However, several lines of evidence argue that this cDNA is an artifact of the cloning procedure and is not a natural gene product. First, we have independently cloned and sequenced 10 cDNAs encoding LAM-1 from both lymphocytes and neutrophils and have found only a single nucleotide sequence with eight single-base polymorphisms (Ord *et al.*, 1990). Second, the enzyme PI-PLC, which specifically cleaves PI-linked proteins, does not affect the level of LAM-1 on lymphocytes or neutrophils. Third, patients with paroxysmal nocturnal hemoglobinuria, a disease characterized in part by the complete absence of PI-linked proteins, display normal levels of serologically and biochemically indistinguishable LAM-1 on all classes of leukocytes. Fourth, the splicing event required to generate this unique cDNA would link two exons in regions that do not contain consensus splice sequences and would thus require a heretofore unknown splicing mechanism. Finally, although two species of LAM-1 mRNA of ≈1.7 and 2.6 kb are expressed by leukocytes (Tedder *et al.*, 1989), we have demonstrated that these two species differ in length within the 3′ untranslated region as a result of differential usage of poly(A) attachment signal sequences. We, therefore, conclude that only a single major species of protein is encoded by the *lyam-1* gene.

C. Structure of the LAM-1 Protein

The LAM-1 protein isolated from lymphocytes has an apparent M_r of ~74,000 after reduction and 68,000 under nonreducing conditions (Tedder *et al.*, 1990b), whereas that of neutrophils is higher, 90,000 to 100,000 after reduction (Griffin *et al.*, 1990). Because the LAM-1 cDNA can only encode ~37 kd of protein, this suggests that the cell surface form of LAM-1 is heavily glycosylated or may undergo additional posttranslational processing. It seems likely that the difference in M_r between different leukocytes is more a reflection of differences in the way different cell types process cell surface molecules, because neutrophils exhibit higher M_r forms of a number of cell surface molecules, including the CD11/CD18 adhesion proteins, CD44 and others. Also, a panel of mAb that identify 16 distinct epitopes of the LAM-1 protein (Spertini *et al.*, 1991c) with many defining functional regions of the protein do not distinguish between different leukocyte types, suggesting that the LAM-1 protein product expressed in several cell types is identical. Therefore, it is unlikely that the differences in posttranslational modification characteristic of different leukocyte lineages play a significant role in directing the distinct patterns of leukocyte migration. Nonetheless, the human protein also migrates with a M_r ~20 kd less than the mouse protein, so further detailed biochemical analysis will be required to determine the nature of these differences.

The cytoplasmic domain of LAM-1 contains two potential sites for phosphorylation (KK*S*KR*S*) by protein kinase C. One of these Ser residues is also conserved in the MEL-14 antigen (KK*S*QER). This potential site for phosphorylation is also encoded by a distinct exon (IX). However, while functional studies of LAM-1 would suggest that it is the target of a kinase, a direct biochemical demonstration of phosphorylation has been difficult, because agents that stimulate phosphorylation also enhance LAM-1 shedding from the cell surface. Most likely, this issue will have to be resolved by transfection of cells with LAM-1 cDNAs containing site specific mutations with subsequent functional analysis.

III. LAM-1 Expression

After the isolation of LAM-1 cDNAs, monoclonal antibodies were developed against the recombinant protein and used to examine the cellular expression of LAM-1. Surprisingly, the anti-LAM-1 antibodies had a pattern of reactivity similar to that previously described for the anti-TQ1 and anti-Leu-8 antibodies (Tedder *et al.*, 1990a; Reinherz *et al.*, 1982; Gatenby *et al.*, 1982), and these antibodies reacted with LAM-1 cDNA transfected cells (Tedder *et al.*, 1990a). Independently, others cloned the Leu-8 antigen and showed that it was identical to LAM-1 (Camerini *et al.*, 1989). The anti-TQ1 and Leu-8 antibodies had previously been used to determine the functional capacity of helper T cell subpopulations that expressed these antigens (Reinherz *et al.*, 1982; Gatenby *et al.*, 1982; Kansas *et al.*, 1985b). Because the terms TQ1 and Leu-8 were initially used to describe the monoclonal antibodies, we have retained the term LAM-1 to describe this receptor in functional terms. Others, however, have subsequently begun to refer to this receptor the DREG antigen (Kishimoto *et al.*, 1990) and LEC-CAM-1 (Stoolman and Ebling, 1989).

The expression of LAM-1 is limited to hematopoietic cells. However, cellular expression is a complex function of lineage, stage of differentiation, activation status, and anatomic location of the cells.

A. LAM-1 Expression by T Lymphocytes and NK Cells

Although LAM-1 can be detected on a significant proportion of thymocytes by flow cytometry, the expression of LAM-1 during T cell ontogeny is complex (Fig. 2). The level of LAM-1 expressed by thymocytes is variable and is generally lower than that found on circulating T cells (Tedder *et al.*, 1990a; Picker *et al.*, 1990). LAM-1^{hi} thymocytes include the $CD3^{bright}$ population, which by several criteria (i.e., $CD4^+$ or 8^+, $CD1^-$, TCR^+, $CD5^{bright}$) include the most mature cells. Interestingly, however, LAM-1 is also detected on a subset of the least mature thymic lymphocytes, although at generally lower levels. Expression of LAM-1 by immature thymocytes may indicate that precursor T cells migrating into the thymus may be LAM-1^+, with LAM-1 expression being differentially regulated during further maturation.

In the periphery, the majority of T cells are uniformly LAM-1^+ (Tedder

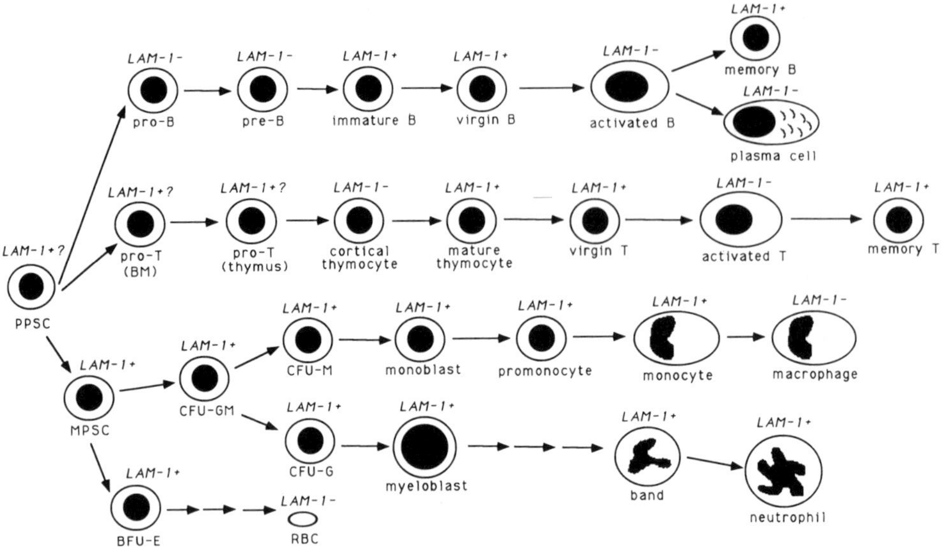

FIGURE 2

Expression of LAM-1 during leukocyte maturation and differentiation. The expression of LAM-1 is depicted during the differentiation of B cells, T cells, neutrophils, and monocytes. As discussed in the text, LAM-1 is expressed late in B cell development, is lost after activation, and is reexpressed on memory cells. A similar pattern holds for T cells, except that LAM-1 may be expressed on committed prothymocytes in the bone marrow (BM) and on early T cell precursors immediately after entry into the thymus. However, LAM-1 expression is low or negative on most common cortical thymocytes (CD1+, $CD3^{lo/-}$), but is expressed on all or most mature thymocytes ($CD3^{hi}$ CD4or8+). LAM-1 is expressed on virgin T cells, is lost after activation, and is reexpressed by most memory T cells. CFU-GM and BFU-E both express LAM-1, implying that their immediate precursor (MPSC) is also $LAM\text{-}1^+$. The LAM-1 phenotype of earlier hematopoietic stem cells is uncertain. Both neutrophil and monocyte precursors express LAM-1 throughout development, whereas LAM-1 expression is lost subsequent to commitment to erythroid development. PPSC, pluripotent stem cell; MPSC, multipotent stem cell; CFU, colony forming unit; M, monocyte; G, granulocyte, RBC, red blood cell. Pro-B and pre-B cells are CD10+ B cell precursors.

et al., 1990a,b). However, distinct subpopulations of both $CD4^+$ and $CD8^+$ cells are $LAM\text{-}1^-$ or express only low levels of LAM-1. We and others have previously used differential expression of LAM-1 to identify helper T lymphocyte ($CD4^+$) subpopulations with different functional properties (Reinherz *et al.,* 1982; Gatenby *et al.,* 1982; Kansas *et al.,* 1985b). Most of the $CD4^+LAM\text{-}1^+$ cells are of the $CD4^+CD45RA^+CD29(VLA\text{-}4)^{lo}$ phenotype that identifies "virgin" or "naive" T cells that do not proliferate in response to soluble antigen (Tedder *et al.,* 1985). However, many (30 to 50%) of the

$CD4^+LAM\text{-}1^+$ cells are of the $CD4^+CD45RA^-CD29^{hi}$ subpopulation of"memory" T cells (Tedder *et al.*, 1990b; Tedder *et al.*, 1985). In studies using purified subpopulations of LAM-1^+ or LAM-1^- memory T helper cells, the majority of B cell help for immunoglobulin secretion was provided by the LAM-1^+ cells, which induced 3 to 7 fold higher levels of secreted Lg than LAM-1^- memory helper T cells (Tedder *et al.*, 1990b). In addition, and most significantly, memory helper T cells expressing LAM-1 generated a significantly stronger proliferative response to tetanus toxoid than those lacking LAM-1 expression. Therefore, both LAM-1^+ and LAM-1^- cells can be found within the CD4 memory cell population, but these two populations exhibit distinct functional profiles.

Some of the surface antigen heterogeneity of memory helper T cells is likely to result from the cells being at different stages of activation or maturation. Consistent with this, prolonged mitogen stimulation of blood lymphocytes results in decreased expression of LAM-1 on the cell surface (Kanof and James, 1988; Tedder *et al.*, 1990a). This would suggest that the most activated helper T cells would be LAM-1^-. However, because LAM-1 can be reexpressed after removal of mitogen stimulation (Kanof and James, 1988), the reexpression of LAM-1 *in vivo* may mark the emergence of antigen specific memory cells. The LAM-1^+ memory cells in blood may represent antigen stimulated cells that have left their sites of initial triggering and have subsequently reacquired expression of LAM-1. The reacquisition of LAM-1 expression would be important in the recruitment of memory cells to sites of inflammation, as well as in the normal recirculation of these cells. Mature lymphocytes can thus alternate between a LAM-1^+ and LAM-1^- phenotype, depending on their activation status and stage of differentiation. The regulated expression of LAM-1 by functionally distinct subpopulations of lymphocytes could also help explain why different lymphocyte subsets show marked differences in their distribution between blood and the afferent and efferent lymph of peripheral lymph nodes (Mackay *et al.*, 1990).

LAM-1 is also expressed by a subpopulation of NK cells (Tedder *et al.*, 1990a). These cells, however, are rarely found in peripheral lymph nodes. The function of LAM-1 on this cell lineage remains uncharacterized. It is possible that LAM-1 may, at least in part, mediate NK cell localization into skin or mucosal epithelium.

B. LAM-1 Expression by B Lymphocytes

LAM-1 is expressed late in B cell ontogeny, after surface IgM expression is achieved, and its expression is tightly coordinated with that of CD44 (Kansas and Dailey, 1989). Virgin, immunocompetent B cells are uniformly

LAM-1$^+$, but as with T cells, LAM-1 expression is lost after mitogenic or antigenic stimulation *in vitro.* Consistent with this observation, germinal center B cells, which constitute a population of actively proliferating and differentiating B cells, are uniformly LAM-1$^-$ (Kansas *et al.,* 1985a). This loss of LAM-1 from activated B cells is reversible, however, because at least some memory B cells are LAM-1$^+$. Among peripheral blood B cells, LAM-1$^-$ B cells include the PWM responsive subset, whereas LAM-1$^+$ B cells are preferentially responsive to *Staphylococcus aureus* Cowan 1. LAM-1 is, therefore, also an important marker for maturational and functional subsets of human B lymphocytes.

C. LAM-1 Expression by Tissue Lymphocytes

LAM-1 is expressed at dramatically higher frequencies and levels by blood lymphocytes when compared with lymphocytes isolated from thymus, bone marrow, and spleen (Tedder *et al.,* 1990a). These differences may relate to the finding that prolonged mitogen stimulation of blood lymphocytes results in decreased expression of LAM-1 on the cell surface (Kanof and James, 1988; Tedder *et al.,* 1990a). Alternatively, lymphocyte entry into lymphoid tissues may directly result in the partial or total loss of LAM-1 from the cell surface. LAM-1 expression by spleen lymphocytes increases dramatically in a subpopulation of the cells after culture, demonstrating that the lower levels of LAM-1 on a subpopulation of spleen lymphocytes is reversible (Tedder *et al.,* 1990a). Thus, there may be an ongoing *in vivo* process in lymphoid tissues that down-regulates LAM-1 expression, but with entry into the circulation and removal of that influence, a subpopulation of these cells may again express LAM-1. The CD45RA$^-$CD29^{hi} T cells in blood that do not express LAM-1 may represent cells that have recently migrated from secondary lymphoid tissues and thus still express only low levels of LAM-1. Decreased expression of LAM-1 may be a general property of tissue or activated lymphocytes because intestinal lamina propria T cells have diminished LAM-1 (Kanof *et al.,* 1988). Most of the T cells in the lungs of sarcoidosis patients lack LAM-1 (Gerli *et al.,* 1989), as do T cells found in synovial fluid (Goto *et al.,* 1987) and biopsy specimens of mycosis fungoides (Abel *et al.,* 1985).

D. LAM-1 Expression by Myelomonocytic Cells and Cells of Other Lineages

Among myeloid cells, LAM-1 is expressed by nearly all circulating neutrophils, monocytes, and eosinophils (Griffin *et al.,* 1990; Tedder *et al.,* 1990a). Monocytes and neutrophils express similar levels of cell surface

LAM-1 as lymphocytes, but activation of these cell types during their isolation usually induces some loss of the molecule from the cell surface. However, neutrophils and monocytes express lower levels of LAM-1 mRNA than lymphocytes, suggesting that message stability or protein processing may be different in myelomonocytic cells (Tedder *et al.*, 1989; Ord *et al.*, 1990). The major portion of LAM-1 is found on the cell surface, and LAM-1 does not appear to localize, to a significant extent, in intracellular compartments.

LAM-1 is expressed more or less continuously throughout myeloid differentiation in the bone marrow (Griffin *et al.*, 1990; Kansas *et al.*, 1990). Whether or not LAM-1 is expressed on the earliest hematopoietic stem cells is not known, but committed myeloid progenitor cells at all levels of maturation are LAM-1$^+$. This includes >80% of CFU-GM, which are the earliest progenitor cell committed to granulocyte/macrophage differentiation. Early erythroid progenitor cells (BFU-E) are also LAM-1$^+$, despite the lack of LAM-1 expression on more mature nucleated and nonnucleated erythrocytes. LAM-1 is also absent from circulating platelets. The role of LAM-1 in the localization or development of progenitor cells is not currently known. Because progenitor cell traffic into lymph nodes or into inflammatory sites is not known to occur, it is possible that LAM-1 may mediate leukocyte/endothelial interactions within the bone marrow. Thus, LAM-1 may play a broader role in cellular movement than was originally realized and may also play an important role in stem cell traffic.

E. Expression of LAM-1 by Malignant Leukocytes

The specific adhesion of some tumor cells to capillary endothelium and the existence of organ specific metastasis suggests that interactions between tumor cells and normal tissues may influence tumor localization. Although the molecules that mediate these events in malignant cells have not been completely described, cell surface molecules involved in the adhesion and migration of normal leukocytes may also be involved in the dissemination of hematopoietic malignancies (Sher *et al.*, 1988). The expression of LAM-1 is most frequently demonstrated in chronic lymphocytic leukemias (CLL) and follicular or diffuse small cleaved cell lymphomas, whereas most other lymphoid malignancies are LAM-1$^-$ (Spertini *et al.*, 1991a). CLL cells rarely express adhesion molecules other than LAM-1, with the exception of CD44. In our studies, greater than 90% of malignancies are CD44$^+$, consistent with its ubiquitous distribution on normal hematopoietic cells. Similar results have been obtained in previous studies of Leu-8 and TQ1 antigen expression by CLL and nonHodgkins lymphomas (Carbone *et al.*, 1988; Strickler *et al.*, 1988; Spertini *et al.*, 1991a). Thus, malignancies that are associated with circulating tumor cells are most likely to be LAM-1^+. However, some CLL cases fail to express LAM-1. Similarly, acute myelomonocytic leukemia and chronic myelogenous leukemia cells rarely expressed LAM-1, in contrast to LAM-1 expression by their normal cellular counterparts. In addition, the frequency and level of LAM-1 expression did not correlate with the tissue source of the malignant cells. Because the expression of LAM-1 is somewhat restricted among hematologic malignancies, the expression, or the absence of expression, may have a major impact on the trafficking of leukemic cells and the dissemination of non-Hodgkins lymphomas into peripheral lymph nodes.

IV. Regulation of LAM-1 Expression

A. LAM-1 Is Shed from the Cell Surface

One interesting and unique feature of the regulation of LAM-1 expression is the loss of this molecule from the surface of leukocytes following cellular activation. Treatment of leukocytes with phorbol esters (PMA) significantly reduces the level of cell surface LAM-1 expressed by blood T and B lymphocytes in less than 30 minutes (Tedder *et al.*, 1990a). Incubating blood lymphocytes overnight at 4°C can also result in a complete loss of LAM-1 from the cell surface (Tedder *et al.*, 1985). This loss actually results from the release or shedding of the molecule (Kishimoto *et al.*, 1990; Spertini *et al.*, 1991a). A large fragment of LAM-1 (M_r 69,000) can be immunoprecipitated from the supernatant fluid of normal lymphocytes cultured with PMA (Spertini *et al.*, 1991a). The quantity of immunoprecipitable protein is essentially identical to the amount that can be immunoprecipitated from detergent solubilized cells, indicating that the major portion, if not all, of the protein is released into the supernatant fluid. That LAM-1 expression is down-modulated by shedding rather than by internalization suggests that a PMA sensitive regulatory pathway, which is distinct from that which regulates down-modulation of most other surface molecules including CD4, controls the expression of LAM-1. A small amount of this soluble isoform of LAM-1 can also be immunoprecipitated from the supernatant fluid of lymphocytes cultured without stimulation suggesting that LAM-1 may be constitutively shed at a slow rate with its expression kept constant by the continuous synthesis of new receptors.

Although the mechanism of shedding is unknown, it does not appear to result from the activation induced secretion of a soluble protease. This is demonstrated in mixing experiments by the observation that neutrophils activated with GM-CSF lose LAM-1, while cell surface expression of LAM-1 by T cells present in the cultures is unaffected. In addition, supernatant fluid from cells that have shed LAM-1 do not contain soluble proteases that can alter cell surface expression of LAM-1. Therefore, it is likely that enzymatic cleavage of this cell surface receptor may result from the specific activation of a membrane bound protease. Alternatively, activation induced changes in the conformation of the LAM-1 protein may expose nascent sites on LAM-1 that are then susceptible to cleavage by soluble proteases. Nonetheless, the finding that all cell lines transfected with LAM-1 cDNAs, including human erythroleukemia cells, mouse fibroblast and pre-B cell lines, and all LAM-1$^+$ malignancies, rapidly modulate LAM-1 after PMA exposure suggests that the protease that cleaves LAM-1 is ubiquitous in distribution (Spertini *et al.*, 1991a).

The activation of protein kinase C may be one biochemical pathway by which the shedding of LAM-1 is regulated, because PMA directly activates protein kinase C. In addition, inhibitors of protein kinase C inhibit PMA induced shedding (Spertini *et al.*, 1991a). This observation directly implicates the conserved Ser residue within the cytoplasmic tail of LAM-1 as a potential site for phosphorylation. Because the shed LAM-1 protein appears intact, except for a loss of M_r of 3000 to 5000, it is likely that the molecule is cleaved at or near the cell surface. This may explain why this region of the molecule is nearly identical between the human and mouse proteins. It will be interesting to determine whether or not the unique level of conservation of this exon is preserved among all LAM-1$^+$ animal species.

B. Lymphocyte Activation Induces LAM-1 Shedding

Lymphocytes exhibit a reversible down-regulation of LAM-1 expression in response to a variety of mitogens (Tedder *et al.*, 1990a). Concomitant with the decrease in LAM-1 expression following PMA treatment, expression of the CD2, CD18 and CD11a adhesion molecules increases, while expression of CD44 is unaffected. Similarly, mitogen stimulation of lymphocytes promotes the gradual loss of LAM-1 from the cell surface, while the levels of expression of CD2, LFA-1, and LFA-3 increase (Sanders *et al.*, 1988; Tedder *et al.*, 1990a). The decrease in LAM-1 expression following mitogen stimulation is almost the reciprocal of the increased expression of the VLA adhesion molecules that appear 2 to 4 weeks after *in vitro* stimulation of lymphocytes, except that LAM-1 expression overlaps to some extent with expression of CD29, the beta chain of the VLA family (Hemler, 1988; Tedder *et al.*, 1990a). Thus, during activation, there appears to be an inverse relationship between the high levels of LAM-1 expression and the expression of other adhesion molecules. The loss of LAM-1 expression following lymphocyte activation *in vivo* with the concomitant increase in expression of CD2, CD18, and CD11a may result in transient but significant changes in the ability of cells to recognize endothelial cell surfaces. This may be a logical occurrence since LAM-1 may mediate leukocyte binding to endothelium prior to entry into secondary lymphoid tissues. Following binding of cells to endothelium, LAM-1 expression may be significantly down-modulated with concomitant increases in expression of other adhesion molecules that may function to retain the cells in the proper lymphoid tissues following activation.

The expression of LAM-1 after activation or tissue localization is likely to be regulated at multiple levels. While activation of lymphocytes with phytohemagglutinin for 18 hours does not result in significant changes in cell surface LAM-1 expression, it does induce an increase in LAM-1 mRNA levels (Tedder *et al.*, 1989). Therefore, it is likely that increased LAM-1 synthesis compensates for shedding and that the level of cell surface expression of LAM-1 is partly a function of the rates of mRNA and protein synthesis. Shedding of LAM-1 is also likely to be responsible for the lower level of LAM-1 expression characteristic of lymphocytes within lymphoid organs. The shedding of LAM-1 after cellular activation is consistent with early observations of Woodruff and colleagues, who recovered a soluble factor from rat lymph that was able to inhibit lymphocyte binding to HEV (Chin *et al.*, 1984; Chin *et al.*, 1980). A further understanding of the concomitant regulation of LAM-1 mRNA and protein synthesis and shedding will be required to fully understand how this molecule regulates leukocyte migration.

C. Neutrophil Activation Induces LAM-1 Shedding

Similar to lymphocytes, neutrophils and monocytes shed LAM-1 following activation, and the time course of shedding by neutrophils is as rapid as PMA induced shedding in lymphocytes. Neutrophil activation by GM-CSF, PMA, LPS, and calcium ionophore all induce LAM-1 shedding. Similar to what is seen in T cells, this decrease in LAM-1 expression is accompanied by a several fold increase in CD11b surface expression (Griffin *et al.*, 1990). The down-regulation of LAM-1 and the up-regulation of CD11b occur simultaneously, with measurable changes seen in 5 minutes and maximum effects at 60 minutes. Interestingly, G-CSF also activates neutrophils but does not induce a loss of LAM-1 *in vitro.* Monocytes also lose LAM-1 following activation, and even simple adherence to plastic at 37°C causes a complete loss of LAM-1 from the cell surface.

As discussed earlier, myeloid progenitor cells express LAM-1, and GM-CSF exposure *in vitro* also induces shedding of the receptor from the surface of these cells (Griffin *et al.*, 1990). In this context, it is noteworthy that GM-CSF also causes profound alterations in the marrow and blood progenitor cell compartments *in vivo* (Socinski *et al.*, 1988). Patients receiving GM-CSF develop rapid and dramatic myeloid hyperplasia in the marrow, but surprisingly, the number of progenitor cells in the marrow decreases. In contrast, the concentration of progenitor cells per milliliter of blood may increase 10 to 100 fold. Thus, it is possible that GM-CSF induced shedding of LAM-1 and changes in other adhesion molecules may contribute to the relocation of progenitor cells from the marrow into the blood. Further characterization of the role of LAM-1 in progenitor cell migration and localization is warranted.

GM-CSF induced shedding of LAM-1 with the concomitant increase in CD11b expression is likely to be a clinically important physiologic response. Exposure of neutrophils to GM-CSF in culture rapidly induces neutrophil aggregation mediated by increased CD11b expression (Arnout *et al.*, 1986). *In vivo,* neutrophils disappear from the circulation approximately 15 to 30 minutes after infusion of GM-CSF (Devereux *et al.*, 1987; Socinski *et al.*, 1988; Peters *et al.*, 1988). This fall in neutrophil concentration is temporally correlated with increased expression of CD11b. Studies with labeled neutrophils suggest that they are trapped in the pulmonary microvasculature, as a result of their large size or due to neutrophil/endothelial interactions (Socinski *et al.*, 1988; Devereux *et al.*, 1987). Surprisingly, 60 to 90 minutes after GM-CSF administration, the number of neutrophils in the blood begins to increase rapidly, despite continued high level expression of CD11b (Socinski *et al.*, 1988). It is noteworthy that migration of human neutrophils into skin windows is also markedly diminished in patients receiving GM-CSF. Interestingly, G-CSF does not induce loss of LAM-1 *in vitro* and does not appear to affect the migration of neutrophils into a skin window (Toner *et al.*, 1989).

Clinical trials using G-CSF and GM-CSF are currently being carried out by Drs George Demetri and James Griffin at the DFCI, affording the ability to examine the relationship between alterations in LAM-1 expression and changes in neutrophil migration (Demetri *et al.*, 1990). Within 1 hour of administration, GM-CSF induced complete shedding of LAM-1 from the neutrophil surface that persisted for up to 6 days *in vivo.* In contrast, G-CSF administration induces a rapid decay in LAM-1 expression that returns to near normal levels within an hour with no sustained effect on the long-term expression of LAM-1. LAM-1⁻ neutrophils would be expected to have an impaired ability to exit from the vascular system, and this could contribute to the observed differential effects of GM-CSF and G-CSF on skin window migration. Studies by others have shown that this acute neutropenia also occured in a patient with leukocyte adhesion deficiency who, therefore, lacks CDllb/CD18 (Yong *et al.*, 1990). These *in vitro* and *in vivo* observations further support the possibility that certain effects of GM-CSF and G-CSF on neutrophil mobility are due to alterations in expression or function of LAM-1.

V. LAM-1 Mediates Lymphocyte Binding to HEV

A. HEV Binding

As mentioned above, cDNA cloning indicates that LAM-1 is the structural homologue of the mouse lymph node homing receptor identified by the MEL-14 antibody. Indirect evidence for a functional homology was obtained by the demonstration that PMA-treated lymphocytes lost both LAM-1 expression and their ability to bind to human peripheral lymph node HEV in the *in vitro* frozen section assay (Tedder *et al.*, 1990a). Furthermore, LAM-1$^+$ CLL cells and lymphoblastoid cell lines bind peripheral node HEV at levels proportional to the amount of LAM-1 expressed, and LAM-1$^-$ CLL cells and lymphoblastoid cell lines do not bind to HEV in this assay (Spertini *et al.*, 1991a). Direct confirmation of this function for LAM-1 was obtained by demonstrating that mAb directed against appropriate epitopes of the LAM-1 molecule inhibit (85 to 90%) the binding of lymphocytes or lymphoid cell lines to rat peripheral lymph node HEV (Kishimoto *et al.*, 1990; Spertini *et al.*, 1991a,b), whereas mAb directed against other epitopes of LAM-1 or other cell surface molecules are without effect (Table I). Studies by Rosen and colleagues have previously shown that Ca^{++} is required for lymphocyte/HEV interactions, consistent with the finding that EDTA can completely abrogate LAM-1 mediated binding (Stoolman *et al.*, 1984; Spertini *et al.*, 1991a,b). It is also likely that the carbohydrate epitope on the ligand expressed by HEV contains sialic acid as intravenously injected sialidase inactivates attachment sites for lymphocytes on HEV (Rosen *et al.*, 1985; Rosen *et al.*, 1989). These data firmly establish that LAM-1 is the adhesion protein critical for lymphocyte binding to peripheral lymph node HEV. Although other adhesion receptors are likely to function as accessory receptors in lymphocyte binding to

TABLE I

The Anti-LAM-1 Monoclonal Antibodies

Name	Staining[a] intensity	HEV[b] binding	PPME[c] binding	Domain[d] binding
TQ1	++	N	wB	L
Leu-8	+++	N	N	L
LAM1-1	+++	B 70%	E	EGF
LAM1-2	++	B 60%	wB	L
LAM1-3	++++	B 85%	B	L
LAM1-4	+++	B 90%	B	L
LAM1-5	+++	N	E	EGF
LAM1-6	+	B 90%	N	L
LAM1-7	++	B 25%	N	L
LAM1-8	+++	N	N	L
LAM1-9	+++	N	N	L
LAM1-10	+++	N	N	L
LAM1-11	+++	N	N	L
LAM1-12	+++	N	N	L
LAM1-13	+	N	N	n.d.
LAM1-14	+++	N	N	SCR
LAM1-15	++	N	N	EGF
LAM1-16	+	N	N	n.d.

[a]The reactivity of leukocytes with anti-LAM-1 monoclonal antibodies were determined by indirect immunofluorescence analysis with the relative intensity of fluorescence staining indicated by a – (no reactivity) to ++++ (highest reactivity) scale.
[b]The ability of each mAb to inhibit lymphocyte binding to HEV. B = blocks binding, E = enhances binding, N = no effect on binding, w = weak effect.
[c]The ability of each mAb to inhibit PPME binding to human lymphocytes.
[d]Binding of the antibodies to domains of LAM-1; L = lectin, EGF or SCR, n.d. = not determined.

HEV, LAM-1 appears to be the dominant adhesion protein mediating human lymphocyte binding (Fig. 3). However, it is certainly likely that adhesion molecules in addition to LAM-1 and LFA-1 are involved in leukocyte entry into inflamed lymph nodes.

B. Regulation of LAM-1 Binding Activity

An important emerging paradigm relevant to all leukocyte adhesion proteins is the multiplicity of mechanisms by which the action of adhesion molecules can be regulated. The first mechanism is via the level of expression. Although LAM-1 does not exhibit distinct levels of expression (i.e., low/hi), as do a number of the integrins, lymphocytes can alternate between LAM-1^+ and LAM-1^- phenotypes, as outlined above. The second

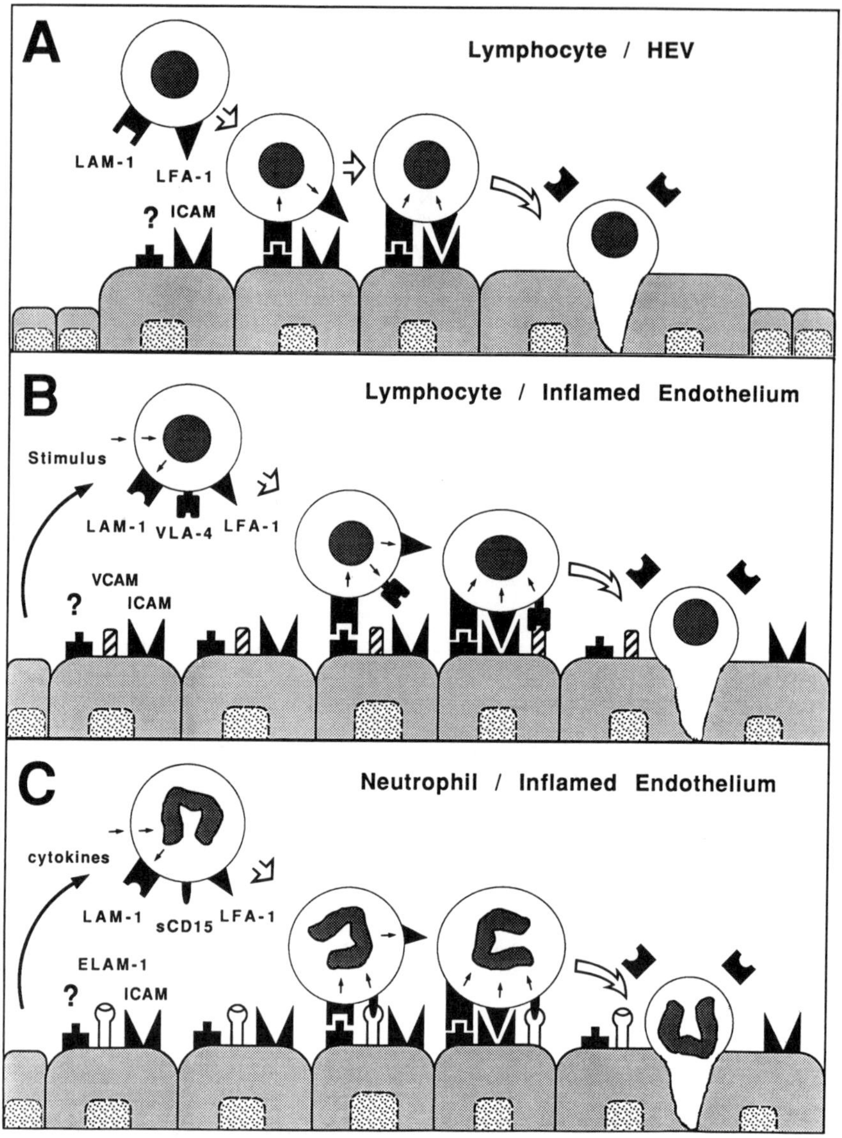

FIGURE 3

Proposed model for the molecular events that regulate lymphocyte binding to HEV (A), and lymphocyte (B) and neutrophil (C) binding to endothelium at sites of inflammation.

mechanism is via the regulation of expression of the ligand(s) for a given adhesion molecule. In this regard, the ligand for LAM-1 appears to be constitutively expressed on HEV of lymph nodes, and a functionally indistinguishable ligand is induced by certain cytokines on endothelial cell monolayers (See following discussion).

The third mechanism by which the activity of an adhesion protein can be regulated is the activation of the molecule itself, usually as a result of cellular activation. Activation of T lymphocytes by cross-linking the CD3/TCR complex or through the CD2 pathway induces a rapid and transient increase in HEV binding that is completely blocked by anti-LAM-1 antibodies (Spertini *et al.*, 1991b). Extensive studies by Rosen and colleagues have shown that a major component of the LAM-1/MEL-14 ligand is carbohydrate in nature and that LAM-1/ligand interactions can be blocked by specific mannose-6 phosphate rich sugars (Stoolman *et al.*, 1984; Yednock *et al.*, 1987a,b). Therefore, the increase in LAM-1 ligand binding activity can also be studied using PPME, the soluble mannan core derived from the yeast *Hansenula holstii,* which binds specifically to LAM-1 (and MEL-14) and defines the lectin specificity of these molecules (Yednock *et al.*, 1987a). PPME is particularly useful for these studies, because it can be labeled with fluorescent or radioactive tags, and its binding can then be studied free of the influence of other adhesion proteins. Using fluorescein labeled PPME, it is possible to demonstrate that neutrophil activation with G-CSF, GM-CSF, or TNFα also induces a significant and transient increase in LAM-1 activity and that activated lymphocytes were similarly able to bind higher amounts of labeled PPME.

The increase in ligand binding activity for lymphocytes and neutrophils peaks at approximately 5 minutes when the cells are stimulated at 37°C and rapidly declines to baseline levels thereafter. This increase in PPME binding does not result from an increase in receptor number. When the cells are stimulated at 4°C, a temperature where many signal transduction pathways, including protein kinase C, remain operable, the increase in binding peaks between 15 to 30 minutes and declines to baseline levels between 1 to 2 hours. Little shedding occurs at 4°C, indicating that this temperature is actually optimal for examining the effects on LAM-1 binding activity. Moreover, LFA-1 mediated binding does not occur at 4°C, suggesting that the signals that activate LAM-1 are distinct from those that activate LFA-1 (Spertini *et al.*, 1991b; Dustin and Springer, 1989). Scatchard analysis of PPME binding activity, using ^{125}I-labeled PPME, demonstrates that increased ligand binding activity results directly from a 4 to 17 fold increase in the affinity of the receptor for ligand. It seems likely that the affinity change for the natural ligand would be even higher and that at

37°C the increase in ligand binding activity is likely to occur within minutes of stimulation, if not sooner.

It is important to note that the cellular activation signals that lead to the increase in affinity of LAM-1, in most cases, are the same signals that lead to the shedding of the molecule. The two processes, however, exhibit different kinetics, with the up-regulation of affinity being much more rapid (seconds to minutes) and the shedding being somewhat slower (minutes to hours). These considerations are important for delineating the role of LAM-1 in adhesion to endothelium at sites of inflammation, as discussed later. The observation that G-CSF induces an increase in neutrophil LAM-1 affinity for ligand equivalent to that obtained with GM-CSF but does not induce shedding, makes it likely that the neutropenia that results from administration of G-CSF and GM-CSF to patients occurs because of the increase in LAM-1 affinity for ligand and is unrelated to shedding. This observation also indicates that the cellular signalling pathways that induce affinity changes and shedding are distinct at some point. An increase in binding activity for other adhesion proteins has also been thoroughly documented for both the VLA and CD11/CD18 integrins (Dustin and Springer, 1989; Shimizu, 1990) and is also characterized by a transient increase in the avidity of the adhesion protein for ligand. These observations suggest that affinity regulation of LAM-1 by lineage specific signals may account, at least in part, for the clear differences observed in the migration patterns of different leukocyte classes.

C. Domains of LAM-1 That Mediate Ligand Binding

As mentioned previously, considerable functional evidence indicates that the lectin domain of LAM-1 and other SELECTINs is likely to subserve an essential function in adhesion by these molecules. In order to precisely determine which domains of the LAM-1 molecule are involved in adhesion, we have developed a large panel of monoclonal antibodies (mAb) reactive with LAM-1 (See Table I). Functional analysis of the effects of mAb binding on adhesion to HEV and binding of PPME reveals several classes of antibodies (Spertini *et al.*, 1991a,c). One class, including anti-LAM1-3 and -4, completely inhibits both the binding of lymphocytes to HEV and the binding of PPME to LAM-1. These data are quite similar to what is observed in the murine system with the MEL-14 mAb (Yednock *et al.*, 1987b) and further demonstrates that the lectin activity of LAM-1 (and MEL-14) is essential to the adhesive properties of the molecule. In addition, these two mAb completely cross-block each others' binding, and the epitope identified by each antibody is located within the lectin domain. Collectively, these data suggest that these two monoclonal antibodies identify epitopes close to the carbohydrate recognition site of LAM-1. Consistent with the absolute requirement for recognition of carbohydrate in lymphocyte adhesion to peripheral node HEV, no antibodies were found that inhibited PPME binding but not HEV binding.

Analysis of chimeric selectins, in which various domains of CD62 are substituted for those of LAM-1, demonstrates that the binding of PPME requires only the lectin domain of LAM-1; the EGF and SCR domains of LAM-1 are not required (Kansas *et al.*, 1991). However, another monoclonal antibody, anti-LAM1-6, which inhibits lymphocyte adhesion to HEV and maps to the lectin domain, does not block the binding of PPME or anti-LAM1-3 or -4 mAb. This suggests that this mAb binds at or near a site that is required for HEV binding but that is not directly involved in recognition of the carbohydrate portion of the ligand. Several lines of evidence suggest that the EGF domain may be all or part of this putative second ligand binding site. This is supported by the finding that the anti-LAM1-1 mAb, which also inhibits lymphocyte adhesion to HEV, binds to the EGF domain. Similar results have been obtained using antibodies reactive with the Ly-22 epitope of the MEL-14 antigen (Siegelman *et al.*, 1990). Experiments in progress should determine directly whether the EGF domain is required for cell adhesion or if it plays some other, perhaps supportive, role in generating the proper structure for the lectin domain.

An unexpected finding was that the binding of several of the anti-LAM-1 antibodies enhanced PPME binding in a manner similar to that observed with leukocyte activation (Spertini *et al.*, 1991c). The mAb that induce this effect all identify closely linked epitopes on the LAM-1 molecule, suggesting that there is a specific region of the protein that is involved in the up-regulation of LAM-1 affinity. However, the two mAb that induce the strongest increase in PPME binding, anti-LAM1-1 and anti-LAM1-5, differ in one important respect: LAM1-1 maps to the EGF-like domain and inhibits lymphocyte binding to HEV, whereas anti-LAM1-5 maps to the EGF domain and does not affect lymphocyte binding to HEV. The mechanism by which anti-LAM1-1 and anti-LAM1-5 induce an increase in the affinity of LAM-1 for carbohydrate is presently unknown. However, a similar phenomenon has been observed with mAb binding to appropriate epitopes on LFA-1 or VLA-4, which induce homotypic adhesion mediated by LFA-1 or VLA-4, respectively (Bednarczyk and McIntyre, 1990; Keizer *et al.*, 1988). Binding of these mAb may directly induce a conformational change in the adhesion molecule that accounts for the observed "activation" of adhesion. Presumably, this putative change in conformation is identical or highly similar to that which occurs with cellular activation

(Dustin and Springer, 1989; Shimizu *et al.*, 1990). Alternatively, binding of mAb to LAM-1 (or other adhesion proteins) may generate transmembrane signals that induce the activation of adhesion molecules. In this regard, several investigators have demonstrated that binding of mAb to various adhesion proteins can transduce signals to the cell, resulting in lymphokine secretion and other evidence of cellular activation. The delineation of the mechanism(s) responsible for this phenomenon will be important in understanding the regulation of LAM-1 function.

The observation that the anti-LAM1-1 antibody inhibits lymphocyte/HEV binding, yet also enhances PPME binding, suggests a dynamic model of receptor/ligand interactions. If the EGF domain is directly involved in adhesion but is not directly involved in binding of carbohydrate, then binding of the EGF domain to its (presumably protein) receptor might alter the affinity of the lectin domain such that carbohydrate is bound more efficiently. This cooperativity would also lead to a high avidity interaction, an important consideration given the observation that LAM-1 has a low affinity for PPME. A two site model for ligand binding is attractive given the observation that the carbohydrate ligands for the SELECTINs are structurally closely related (Stoolman *et al.*, 1987; Yednock *et al.*, 1987a); a requirement for a second binding site might also confer a higher degree of specificity on the adhesive event. Thus, it is possible that the region of LAM-1 identified by the anti-LAM1-1 mAb is the first portion of the receptor to interact with ligand, and that as a result of this interaction, conformational changes in the molecule occur that induce high affinity interactions between LAM-1 and the carbohydrate portion of the ligand. Identification and biochemical characterization of the ligand for LAM-1 will undoubtedly clarify many of these issues.

VI. LAM-1 Mediates Leukocyte Binding to Endothelium

Several lines of evidence have been presented that suggest LAM-1/MEL-14 plays a critical role in the localization of neutrophils into inflamed tissues. Neutrophil binding to HEV from inflamed lymph nodes is inhibited by MEL-14 antibody, and neutrophils that have lost MEL-14 expression due to activation *in vivo* or *in vitro* do not bind to HEV and do not home to inflammatory sites *in vivo* (Jutila *et al.*, 1989; Lewinsohn *et al.*, 1987). In addition, i.v. administration of MEL-14 antibody inhibits accumulation of neutrophils in inflammatory lesions (Jutila *et al.*, 1989). However, the intravenous or intraperitoneal administration of the MEL-14 antibody, in our hands, results in acute and dramatic changes in the number of neutrophils present in the circulating pool. This does not result from the introduction of contaminating LPS in the antibody preparations, because C3H mice that lack the LPS receptor also undergo this dramatic neutropenia. Therefore, it is possible that MEL-14 antibody binding to circulating neutrophils results in Fc mediated clearance/trapping of the neutrophils.

A. Lymphocyte Binding to Activated Endothelium

We have developed direct evidence that LAM-1 functions in contexts other than lymphocyte binding to lymph node HEV. In particular, the expression of LAM-1 on all leukocyte classes led us to ask whether or not this molecule might play a role in the recruitment of all classes of leukocytes to sites of inflammation. Preliminary experiments demonstrated that anti-LAM-1 mAb had little or no effect on the binding of leukocytes to human umbilical vein endothelial cell (HUVEC) monolayers when these assays are performed under "traditional" conditions. However, when lymphocyte binding to cytokine treated HUVEC was assessed under conditions that approximate those of the classic HEV frozen section assay, anti-LAM-1 mAb consistently inhibit binding. Importantly, the anti-LAM-1 mAb that are inhibitory in this assay are the same as those that are inhibitory in the classic frozen section HEV assay. The binding of lymphocytes mediated by LAM-1 in this assay is completely dependent on the prior activation of the HUVEC with proinflammatory cytokines such as IL-1, LPS and TNF, indicating that the LAM-1 ligand is inducibly expressed on these cells. These data directly demonstrate the presence of a functionally indistinguishable ligand on the surface of activated endothelium, and therefore, support the hypothesis that LAM-1 plays an important role in the recruitment of leukocytes to sites of inflammation *in vivo.*

The precise contribution of LAM-1 to lymphocyte binding to endothelium can be inferred from functional studies where mAb reactive with different adhesion molecules can be used to inhibit binding. When the assay described above is performed at 4°C with peripheral blood lymphocytes, blocking mAb to LAM-1, VLA-4 or VCAM-1 each inhibit binding by ~50%, while the combination of mAb to VLA-4 or VCAM-1 plus mAb to LAM-1 inhibits >90% of binding. Antibodies to other cell surface molecules, including ELAM-1, ICAM-1, CD44, and LFA-1 are without detectable effect. The lack of effect of mAb to LFA-1 is probably due to the temperature requirements of LFA-1/ICAM-1 interactions, because when this assay is performed at 37°C, anti-CD18 mAb inhibit ~30% of lymphocyte binding. Anti-LAM-1 and anti-VLA-4 mAb inhibit 40% and 30%, respectively, when this assay is performed at 37°C and the combination of all three mAb inhibits binding by >90%. Thus, optimal lymphocyte binding to endothelium involves the interactions of multiple adhesion molecules.

B. Neutrophil Binding to Activated Endothelium

Using the assay described above, we have also obtained direct evidence that LAM-1 is an important contributor to neutrophil interactions with activated endothelium. Anti-LAM-1 antibodies inhibit ~50% of neutrophil binding to activated endothelium and anti-ELAM-1 mAb inhibit ~40% of binding when the experiments are carried out at 4°C. The combination of anti-LAM-1 and anti-ELAM-1 antibodies, blocks ≈90% of neutrophil binding. At 37°C, anti-CD18 mAb inhibit ~30% of binding, while anti-LAM-1 and anti-ELAM-1 mAb inhibit 40% and 30% of binding, respectively. The previous failure to detect the LAM-1 dependent component of binding most likely results from the different assay systems used to assess binding. Whether or not this results from the LAM-1 interaction being of low avidity, the continual shedding of LAM-1 at 37°C, a requirement for rotation, or other factors, has yet to be determined. Thus, similar yet distinct combinations of adhesion proteins regulate lymphocyte and neutrophil binding to endothelium, and LAM-1 is used by both classes of leukocytes.

Taken together, these data suggest the following model of leukocyte recruitment during inflammation (Fig. 3, B and C). Proinflammatory cytokines released by cells within inflamed tissues (macrophages, dendritic cells, etc.) induce changes in the surrounding endothelium, including the *de novo* expression of ligands for leukocyte adhesion molecules: ELAM-1, VCAM-1, and the LAM-1 ligand. Adhesion of circulating leukocytes to inflamed endothelium is initiated by LAM-1 binding to its ligand, and this initial interaction is stabilized by interaction of VLA-4 with VCAM-1 (for lymphocytes) (Elices *et al.*, 1990; Freedman *et al.*, 1990) or ELAM-1 with sialylated CD15 (sLe^X/sLNF III) (for neutrophils) (Walz *et al.*, 1990; Phillips *et al.*, 1990). The observation that ELAM-1 expression decays, even in the continued presence of inflammatory stimuli, whereas the expression of both VCAM-1 and the LAM-1 ligand is retained as long as the inflammatory stimulus is present, is consistent with the classic observation that neutrophils initially predominate in response to acute inflammation, whereas mononuclear cells predominate at later time points. Once the adhesion of the leukocyte to the luminal surface of the endothelial cell is stabilized, LAM-1 is proteolytically cleaved from the lymphocyte cell surface, allowing the movement of the leukocyte across the surface of the endothelial cell to endothelial cell–cell junctions. This movement probably relies on a combination of the CD11/CD18 proteins and VLA-4. Leukocyte diapedesis between endothelial cells then ensues, relying on interactions between the CD11/CD18 proteins and their ligands, as well as the action of the other VLA integrins with laminin, fibronectin, collagen, and a series of other constituents of the extracellular matrix. Thus, the sequential and overlapping use of multiple leukocyte adhesion molecules allows for the full range of migratory potential to be exhibited by all classes of leukocytes in the course of host defense. Although the outlines of this scheme are now clear, further research will be required in order to understand how the concerted action of these adhesion molecules is regulated.

VII. Evolutionary Conservation of LAM-1

Previous work by others has established that the properties of lymphocyte binding to peripheral node HEV exhibit a high degree of evolutionary conservation (Stoolman *et al.*, 1987; Wu *et al.*, 1988). Specifically, lymphocytes of human or rodent species bind to human or rodent lymph node HEV using cell surface structures that display indistinguishable sugar specificities, divalent cation requirements, and organ specificity. The observation that the LAM-1 and MEL-14 cDNA sequences are >80% homologous is consistent with this high degree of functional conservation. We have extended these observations of evolutionary conservation by determining the pattern of expression of the epitopes identified by our panel of mAb on a variety of mammalian species. Consistent with the crucial role and conserved specificity of this adhesion molecule, several important functionally defined epitopes were expressed by a variety of animal species. In particular, the LAM1-3 epitope, which appears to be involved in carbohydrate binding and might, therefore, be expected to be the most well conserved, is expressed by every species examined, except for rodent or avian species, which are not recognized by any of these mAb. None of the anti-LAM-1 mAb were restricted in their expression to human cells. In addition, a number of the epitopes defined by the functionally silent mAb were also well conserved, suggesting an important degree of structural conservation that extends to the three dimensional structure of LAM-1.

Functional studies revealed that a variety of heterologous species can bind PPME, and this binding can be inhibited by the appropriate anti-LAM-1 mAb (Spertini *et al.*, 1991c). In addition, the binding of lymphocytes of several species to HEV of rat lymph nodes can also be significantly inhibited by mAb to LAM-1. Both the structure and function of this adhesion molecule have, therefore, been well conserved throughout mammalian evolution, underscoring the crucial importance of this adhesion protein to the proper functioning of the immune system. Finally, it is interesting that chickens, which do not have lymph nodes (Glick, 1982), also do not have a LAM-1 homologue that is detected by this panel of mAb. Given the apparent importance of LAM-1 in recruitment of leukocytes to sites of inflammation, it would be interesting to determine if the chicken has evolved other mechanisms for this function or if the chicken LAM-1 molecule is simply too evolutionarily distant to share any of the epitopes defined by our panel of anti-LAM-1 mAb.

VIII. Conclusions

The identification and molecular cloning of the SELECTINs has resulted in an enormous advance in our understanding of leukocyte migration at both the functional and molecular level. It is clear that these molecules and their ligands, in concert with other adhesion receptors and their ligands, interact to regulate leukocye–endothelial cell interactions and hence the migration patterns of leukocytes. The well-conserved nature of LAM-1 through recent evolution and the lack of an immunodeficiency state characterized by the loss of LAM-1, suggests that they serve a crucial role in the immune response. The present availability of cDNAs, cDNA-transfected cell lines, and mAb reactive with multiple functional epitopes of LAM-1 will further accelerate our understanding of these molecules. A few of the remaining important questions regarding LAM-1 are

1. What is the biochemical nature of the ligand?
2. How is the affinity increase with cellular activation achieved and regulated?
3. What is the function, if any, of the shed isoform of LAM-1 in regulating migration?
4. What is the mechanism of LAM-1 shedding and how is it regulated?

The answers to these questions will undoubtedly have an important impact not only in our understanding of leukocyte adhesion and migration but will have clinical implications as well. A detailed understanding of leukocyte recruitment in inflammation, for example, may allow the design of novel pharmacologic reagents capable of inhibiting the recruitment of cells to the inflammatory lesions characteristic of chronic autoimmune disease, such as rheumatoid arthritis. The demonstrated role of functional endothelial/leukocyte adhesion molecules on tumor cells, including LAM-1 (Spertini *et al.*, 1991a), suggests that metastasis could also be clinically targeted. Undoubtedly, the rapid pace of research in this important area will soon provide those clinical applications.

Acknowledgment

This work was supported by grants from the National Institutes of Health, AI-26872 and CA-34183.

References

Abel, E. A., Wood, G. S., Hoppe, R. T., and Warnke, R. A. (1985). *J. Invest. Dermatol.* **85,** 199–202.

Arnout, M. A., Wang, E. A., Clark, S. C., and Sieff, C. A. (1986). *J. Clin. Invest.* **78,** 597–601.

Bednarczyk, J. L., and McIntyre, B. W. (1990). *J. Immunol.* **144,** 777–784.

Berg, E. L., Goldstein, L. A., Jutila, M. A., Nakache, M., Picker, L. J., Streeter, P. R., Wu, N. W., Zhou, D., and Butcher, E. C. (1989). *Immunol. Rev.* **108,** 5–18.

Bevilacqua, M. P., Stengelin, S., Gimbrone, M. A., Jr., and Seed, B. (1989). *Science* **243,** 1160–1164.

Bowen, B., Nguyen, T., and Lasky, L. A. (1989). *J. Cell Biol.* **109,** 421–427.

Camerini, D., James, S. P., Stamenkovic, I., and Seed, B. (1989). *Nature (London)* **342,** 78–80.

Carbone, A., Manconi, R., Poletti, A., Gloghini, A., De Paoli, P. R., and Volpe, R. (1988). *J. Pathol.* **154,** 133–140.

Chin, Y. H., Carey, G. D., and Woodruff, J. J. (1980). *J. Immunol.* **125,** 1764–1769.

Chin, Y. H., Rasmussen, R., Cakiroglu, A. G., and Woodruff, J. J. (1984). *J. Immunol.* **133,** 2961–2965.

Collins, T., Williams, A., Johnston, G. I., Kim, J., Eddy, R., Shows, T., Gimbrone, M. A., Jr., and Bevilacqua, M. P. (1991). *J. Biol. Chem.* **266,** 2466–2478.

Demetri, G. D., Spertini, O., Pratt, E. S., Kim, E., Elias, A., Antman, K., Tedder, T. F., and Griffin, J. D. (1990). *Blood* **76 (Suppl. 1),** 107a.

Devereux, S., Linch, D. C., Campos Costa, D., Spittle, M. F., and Jelliff, A. M. (1987). *Lancet* **2,** 1523–1524.

Drickamer, K. (1988). *J. Biol. Chem.* **263,** 9557–9560.

Dustin, M. L., and Springer, T. A. (1989). *Nature (London)* **341,** 619–624.

Elices, M. J., Osborn, L., Takada, Y., Crouse, C., Luhowskyj, S., Hemler, M. E., and Lobb, R. R. (1990). *Cell* **60,** 577–584.

Freedman, A. S., Munro, J. M., Rice, G. E., Bevilaqua, M. P., Morimoto, C., McIntyre, B. W., Rhynhar, K., Pober, J., and Nadler, L. M. (1990). *Science* **249,** 1030–1033.

Gallatin, W. M., Weissman, I. L., and Butcher, E. C. (1983). *Nature (London)* **304,** 30–34.

Gatenby, P. A., Kansas, G. S., Xian, C. Y., Evans, R. L., and Engleman, E. G. (1982). *J. Immunol.* **129,** 1997–2000.

Gerli, R., Darwish, S., Broccucci, L., Spinozzi, F., and Rambotti, P. (1989). *Chest* **95,** 811–816.

Glick, B. (1982). In "The Reticuloendothelial System, Phylogeny and Ontogeny" (N. Cohen and M. Sigel, eds.), pp. 509–540. Plenum, New York.

Goldstein, L. A., Zhou, D. F. H., Picker, L. J., Minty, C. N., Bargatze, R. F., Ding, J. F., and Butcher, E. C. (1989). *Cell* **56,** 1063–1072.

Goto, M., Miyamoto, T., Nishioka, K., and Uchida, S. (1987). *Arthritis. Rheum.* **30,** 737–743.

Griffin, J. D., Spertini, O., Ernst, T. J., Belvin, M. P., Levine, H. B., Kanakura, Y., and Tedder, T. F. (1990). *J. Immunol.* **145,** 576–584.

Hemler, M. E. (1988). *Immunol. Today* **9,** 109–113.

Jalkanen, S., Bargatze, R. F., de los Toyos, J., and Butcher, E. C. (1987). *J. Cell. Biol.* **105,** 983–990.

Jalkanen, S., Bargatze, R. F., Herron, L. H., and Butcher, E. C. (1986). *Eur. J. Immunol.* **16,** 1195–1202.

Johnston, G. I., Bliss, G. A., Newman, P. J., and McEver, R. P. (1990). *J. Biol. Chem.* **34,** 21381–21385.

Johnston, G. I., Cook, R. G., and McEver, R. P. (1989). *Cell* **56,** 1033–1044.

Jutila, M. A., Rott, L., Berg, E. L., and Butcher, E. C. (1989). *J. Immunol.* **143,** 3318–3324.

Kanof, M. E., and James, S. P. (1988). *J. Immunol.* **140,** 3701–3706.

Kanof, M. E., Strober, W., Ficchi, C., Zeitz, M., and James, S. P. (1988). *J. Immunol.* **140,** 3029–3036.

Kansas, G. S., and Dailey, M. O. (1989). *J. Immunol.* **142,** 3058–3062.

Kansas, G. S., Muirhead, M. J., and Dailey, M. O. (1990). *Blood* **76,** 2483–2492.

Kansas, G. S., Spertini, O., and Tedder, T. F. (1991). *J. Cell. Biol.* **114,** 351–358.

Kansas, G. S., Wood, G. S., and Engleman, E. G. (1985a). *J. Immunol.* **134,** 3003–3006.

Kansas, G. S., Wood, G. S., Fishwild, D. M., and Engleman, E. G. (1985b). *J. Immunol.* **134,** 2995–3002.

Keizer, G. D., Visser, W., Vliem, M., and Figdor, G. (1988). *J. Immunol.* **141,** 1393–1400.

Kishimoto, T. K., Jutila, M. A., and Butcher, E. C. (1990). *Proc. Natl. Acad. Sci. U.S.A.* **87,** 2244–2248.

Larsen, E., Celi, E. A., Gilbert, G. E., Furie, B. C., Erban, J. K., Bonfanti, R., Wagner, D. D., and Furie, B. (1990). *Cell* **59,** 305–312.

Lasky, L. A., Singer, M. S., Yednock, T. A., Dowbenko, D., Fennie, C., Rodriguez, H., Nguyen, T., Stachel, S., and Rosen, S. D. (1989). *Cell* **56,** 1045–1055.

Lewinsohn, D. M., Bargatze, R. F., and Butcher, E. C. (1987). *J. Immunol.* **138,** 4313–4321.

Mackay, C. R., Marston, W. L., and Dudler, L. (1990). *J. Exp. Med.* **171,** 801–817.

Michie, S. A., Garcia, D. F., Stickler, J. G. F., Dailey, M. O., Rouse, R. V., and Warnke, R. A. (1987). *Am. J. Clin. Pathol.* **88,** 486–490.

Miyake, K., Underhill, C. B., Lesley, J., and Kincade, P. W. (1990). *J. Exp. Med.* **172,** 69–75.

Ord, D. C., Ernst, T. J., Zhou, L. J., Rambaldi, A., Spertini, O., Griffin, J. D., and Tedder, T. F. (1990). *J. Biol. Chem.* **265,** 7760–7767.

Peters, W. P., Stuart, A., Affronti, M. L., Kim, C. S., and Coleman, R. E. (1988). *Blood* **72,** 1310–1315.

Phillips, M. L., Nudelman, E., Gaeta, F. C. A., Perez, M., Singhal, A. K., Hakomori, S.-I., and Paulson, J. C. (1990). *Science* **250,** 1130–1132.

Picker, L., Terstappen, L., Rott, L., Streeter, P., Stein, H., and Butcher, E. (1990). *J. Immunol.* **145,** 3247–3255.

Reinherz, E. L., Morimoto, C., Fitzgerald, K. A., Hussey, R. E., Daley, J. F., and Schlossman, S. F. (1982). *J. Immunol.* **128,** 463–468.

Rosen, S. D., Chi, S. I., True, D. D., Singer, M. S., and Yednock, T. A. (1989). *J. Immunol.* **142,** 1895–1902.

Rosen, S. D., Singer, M. S., Yednock, Y. A., and Stoolman, L. M. (1985). *Science* **228,** 1005–1007.

Sanders, M. E., Makgoba, M. W., Sharrow, S. O., Stephany, D., Springer, T. A., Young, H. A., and Shaw, S. (1988). *J. Immunol.* **140,** 1401–1407.

Sher, B. T., Bargatze, R., Holzman, B., Galatin, W. M., Matthews, D., Wu, N., Picker, L., Butcher, E. C., and Weissman, I. L. (1988). *Adv. Can Res.* **51,** 361–389.
Shimizu, Y., Van Seventer, G. A., Horgan, K. J., and Shaw, S. (1990). *Nature (London)* **345,** 250–255.
Siegelman, M. H., Cheng, I. C., Weissman, I. L., and Wakeland, E. K. (1990). *Cell* **61,** 611–622.
Siegelman, M. H., van de Rijn, M., and Weissman, I. L. (1989). *Science* **243,** 1165–1172.
Siegelman, M. H., and Weissman, I. L. (1989). *Proc. Natl. Acad. Sci. U.S.A.* **86,** 5562–5566.
Socinski, M. A., Cannistra, S. A., Sullivan, R., Elis, A., Antman, K., Schnipper, L., and Griffin, J. D. (1988). *Blood* **72,** 691–697.
Spertini, O., Freedman, A. S., Belvin, M. P., Penta, A. C., Griffin, J. D., and Tedder, T. F. (1991a). *Leukemia* **5,** 300–308.
Spertini, O., Kansas, G. S., Munro, J. M., Griffin, J. D., and Tedder, T. F. (1991b). *Nature (London)* **349,** 691–693.
Spertini, O., Kansas, G. S., Reimann, K. A., Mackay, C. R., and Tedder, T. F. (1991c). *J. Immunol.* (in press).
Springer, T. A. (1990). *Nature (London)* **346,** 425–433.
Stamenkovic, I., Amiot, M., Pesando, J. M., and Seed, B. (1989). *Cell* **56,** 1057–1062.
Stamper, H. B., Jr., and Woodruff, J. J. (1976). *J. Exp. Med.* **144,** 828–833.
Stoolman, L. M. (1989). *Cell* **56,** 907–910.
Stoolman, L. M., and Ebling, H. (1989). *J. Clin. Invest.* **84,** 1196–1205.
Stoolman, L. M., Tenforde, T. S., and Rosen, S. D. (1984). *J. Cell. Biol.* **99,** 1535–1540.
Stoolman, L. M., Yednock, T. A., and Rosen, S. D. (1987). *Blood* **70,** 1842–1850.
Strickler, J. G., Medeiros, L. J., Copenhaver, C. M., Weiss, L. M., and Warnke, R. A. (1988). *Humn. Pathol.* **19,** 550–554.
Tedder, T. F., Cooper, M. D., and Clement, L. T. (1985). *J. Immunol.* **134,** 2989–2994.
Tedder, T. F., Ernst, T. J., Demetri, G. D., Isaacs, C. M., Adler, D. A., and Disteche, C. M. (1989). *J. Exp. Med.* **170,** 123–133.
Tedder, T. F., Penta, A. C., Levine, H. B., and Freedman, A. S. (1990a). *J. Immunol.* **144,** 532–540.
Tedder, T. F., Matsuyama, T., Rothstein, D. M., Schlossman, S. F., and Morimoto, C. (1990b). *Eur. J. Immunol.* **20,** 1351–1355.
Toner, G. C., Jakubowski, A. A., Crown, J. P. L., Meisenberg, B., Sheridan, C., and Gabrilove, J. L. (1989). *Ann. Intern. Med.* **110,** 846–847.
Walz, G., Aruffo, A., Kolanus, W., Bevilacqua, M., and Seed, B. (1990). *Science* **250,** 1132–1134.
Watson, M. L., Kingsmore, S. F., Johnston, G. I., Siegelman, M. H., Le Beau, M. M., Lemons, R. S., Bora, N. S., Howard, T. A., Weissman, I. L., McEver, R. P., and Seldin, M. F. (1990). *J. Exp. Med.* **172,** 263–272.
Wu, N. W., Jalkanen, S., Streeter, P. R., and Butcher, E. C. (1988). *J. Cell. Biol.* **107,** 1845–1851.
Yednock, T. A., Stoolman, L. M., and Rosen, S. D. (1987a). *J. Cell. Biol.* **104,** 713–723.
Yednock, T. A., Butcher, E. C., Stoolman, L. M., and Rosen, S. D. (1987b). *J. Cell. Biol.* **104,** 725–731.
Yednock, T. A., and Rosen, S. D. (1989). *Adv. Immunol.* **44,** 313–378.
Yong, K., Rowles, P., Webster, A. D. B., and Linch, D. C. (1990). *Blood* **76(Suppl. 1),** 199a.

CHAPTER 4

The Peripheral Lymph Node Homing Receptor: Tandem Structural and Functional Domains in a Novel Class of Adhesion Molecule

Mark H. Siegelman* and Irving L. Weissman

Howard Hughes Medical Institute and Laboratory of
Experimental Oncology
Department of Pathology
Stanford University School of Medicine
Stanford, California 94305

I. Introduction

The emergence of a new class of adhesion molecule has occurred in the form of three cell surface molecules with similar protein structures (Bevilacqua *et al.*, 1989; Johnston *et al.*, 1989; Lasky *et al.*, 1989; Siegelman *et al.*, 1989). All three also share functions critical to interactions between circ-

*Present address: Department of Pathology, University of Texas Southwestern Medical Center at Dallas, Dallas, Texas 75235

ulating cells and the vasculature. It is the vascular barrier that must be breeched in the course of normal extravasation of lymphocytes (or other hematolymphoid cells) in order to access antigen and antigen presenting cells in lymphoid organs, in tissues, or both to wall-off or eliminate foreign insult in those tissues. This cellular traffic is responsible for desired and undesired inflammation to proceed when normal cells are involved and for metastasis to occur when the migrating cells are neoplastic. The vessel wall is also the surface at which thrombogenesis occurs. It is becoming clear that members of this new class of adhesion molecule, designated LEC-CAMs (Stoolman, 1989), or SELECTINs (Watson *et al.*, 1990) are distinct from other major classes of adhesion receptor families such as integrins, the immunoglobulin gene superfamily, or cadherins, and are vital participants in all of the above biological processes.

One essential event required for the development of lymphoid organs, and appropriate progression of the immune response, takes place at the interface between a lymphocyte's mobile circulating phase and its relatively sessile phase within a particular lymphoid organ. Continual percolation of lymphocytes through lymphoid organs effectively exposes each to the entire repertoire of antigen-reactive cells. Lymphocytes recirculate from blood to lymphoid organs and back to blood, generally passing via efferent lymphatic vessels and their collecting ducts. The specific portal of entry of lymphocytes from the blood stream into peripheral lymphoid organs was identified as specialized postcapillary venules bearing unusually high-walled endothelia (Gowans and Knight, 1964; Marchesi and Gowans, 1964) and named high endothelial venules (HEVs) (Stamper and Woodruff, 1976). The fundamental role of HEV-lymphocyte interaction in lymphocyte trafficking has been demonstrated (Gutman and Weissman, 1973; Howard *et al.*, 1972). The cell surface structures mediating adherence to HEVs prior to translocation through the vessel wall have been designated lymphocyte homing receptors (Gallatin *et al.*, 1983), and their complementary ligands on the endothelial surface have been called "addressins" (Streeter *et al.*, 1988). Recirculating lymphocytes, but not other blood-borne cells, specifically recognize, adhere to luminal walls, and migrate through this highly specialized endothelium into the lymphoid organ parenchyma. Both B and T lymphocytes enter lymphoid organs via common HEVs (Gutman and Weissman, 1973; Howard *et al.*, 1972; Weissman, 1967; Weissman *et al.*, 1977) and thereafter migrate through fields of antigen presenting cells to T-cell or B-cell domains (Gutman and Weissman, 1971; Gutman and Weissman, 1972; Weissman *et al.*, 1974).

Migration of lymphocytes from blood to lymphoid organs has been shown to occur nonrandomly. Peripheral node lymphocytes exhibit binding preference for peripheral node HEVs, while lymphocytes derived from Peyer's patches bind preferentially to Peyer's patch HEV (Stevens *et al.*,

1982). Studies have confirmed that specificity of homing results from the particular complement of homing receptors actively expressed by any one lymphocyte (Howard *et al.*, 1972; Kraal *et al.*, 1983). Subsequent studies of lymphocyte populations and cell lines showed mutually exclusive homing to either lymph node HEV or Peyer's patch HEV, indicating that the two specificities are mediated by independent cell surface structures. A number of murine lymphomas are unispecific with regard to Peyer's patch or peripheral lymph node HEV binding (Gallatin *et al.*, 1983), while others recognize neither venule type. Therefore, lymphocyte homing appears to be regulated by the expression of complementary adhesion molecules on each of the two participants, the homing receptors on recirculating lymphocytes, and the vascular addressins on specialized particular organ HEVs, providing a powerful influence on the distribution of lymphocytes within an organism. The presence of homing receptors on neoplastic lymphoid cells accurately predicts the lymphoid organs to which they metastasize (Bargatze *et al.*, 1987; Sher *et al.*, 1988).

The structures involved in the HEV recognition process could be approached with the availability of clonal lymphoid cell lines having exclusive specificity for a single HEV type, offering the opportunity to define directly these cell surface molecules. A monoclonal antibody, MEL-14, was developed that detects a cell surface determinant present only on those murine T- and B-cells that bind peripheral lymph node HEVs, but not on those that bind either Peyer's patch HEV only or have no HEV binding activity at all (Gallatin *et al.*, 1983). Additionally, MEL-14 specifically ablated binding of normal or neoplastic cells to peripheral node HEVs. The concordance of these observations suggested that the monoclonal antibody recognized the actual receptor. Cell surface structures implicated in HEV binding have also been identified in other species (Chin *et al.*, 1986; Idzerda *et al.*, 1989; Jalkanen *et al.*, 1987; Jalkanen *et al.*, 1986; Rasmussen *et al.*, 1985; Woodruff *et al.*, 1987). A Peyer's patch-specific lymphocyte homing receptor has been shown to be an α/β heterodimer, LPAM (Holzmann *et al.*, 1989; Holzmann and Weissman, 1989), closely related to the VLA-4 member of the integrin family composed of α_4 and a novel β chain designated β_p. This receptor is discussed in Chapter 5.

II. Protein Characterization of the Mouse Lymph Node Homing Receptor

MEL-14 specifically precipitates from the cell surface of lymph node HEV-binding lymphocytes a protein species with apparent molecular weight of about 90 kd (Gallatin *et al.*, 1983), which we have designated $gp90^{MEL-14}$

(Siegelman *et al.*, 1986). Partial aminoterminal amino acid sequence analysis of this molecule, purified to homogeneity, revealed the presence of two aminotermini, one corresponding to the aminoterminus of the highly conserved polypeptide ubiquitin and the other to a unique sequence representing the core polypeptide of the receptor (Siegelman *et al.*, 1986). These findings, in concert with lambda gt11 screening and epitope mapping studies, lead to a proposed model of the receptor complex as a core polypeptide modified by ubiquitination and extensive glycosylation (Siegelman *et al.*, 1986; St. John *et al.*, 1986). In addition, it was inferred from functional correlates that the region of the site(s) of ubiquitination might participate in the adhesion event. In particular, MEL-14, a functional monoclonal antibody, was determined to recognize a ubiquitin dependent determinant (Siegelman *et al.*, 1986; St. John *et al.*, 1986). It was shown that MEL-14 binds specifically to the carboxyterminal 13 residue peptide of, but not intact, ubiquitin, unless previously denatured in SDS. Additionally, the avidity of binding to the carboxyterminal peptides appeared relatively low compared to antibodies made to intact ubiquitin and recognizing specific peptides. This further suggested that MEL-14 recognizes the carboxyterminus of ubiquitin only as a portion of the entire MEL-14 determinant and that the entire epitope is formed by a conjugate-specific determinant or a conformational alteration distant from the ubiquitin moiety induced by ubiquitin conjugation to the core polypeptide.

Other indirect evidence for the presence of ubiquitin modification of the core polypeptide has accumulated. Two MEL-14 specific species were identified on immunoprecipitation of COS-7 cell cDNA transfectants, differing by about 10 kD (Siegelman *et al.*, 1989). This indicated processing of the transcript into discrete forms, and perhaps reflects alternative pathways of posttranslational modification, including ubiquitination, particularly since the observed molecular weight difference is consistent with the addition of a single ubiquitin moiety (8.5 kd). An additional observation perhaps bearing on the possible site of ubiquitination derives from the features of the sequence of the aminoterminal lectin domain. Particularly intriguing may be the lysine richness of the lectin domain. Between conserved residues Asn82, and Glu88 (the region where the conserved Gly is absent) there is a cluster of three lysine residues and an insertion relative to the consensus sequence of five charged amino acids between Cys17 and Gly24 of the consensus sequence of several related lectins. No other insertions or deletions are required to align this portion of the mLHRc sequence with the consensus sequence of other lectin domains. This portion of the domain in mLHRc contains 10 positively charged residues, 3 Arg and 7 Lys. Comparison to the analogous portion of carbohydrate binding domains of other animal lectins shows rat hepatic lectin-1 (RHL-1) to be the most enriched in basic amino acids with 4 Arg in the same region

```
Consensus  W           P   N             E D C V                               G   W N D       C
hLHRc        W G D G E P N N K K N K E D C V E I Y I K A N K D A G K W N D D A C H K L K A A L
mLHRc        W G A G E P N N K K S K E D C V E I Y I K A E A D S G K W N D D A C H K A K A A L

IgEr hu      W A P G E P T S A S Q G E D C V M M - - - - - - A G S G A W N D A F C D A K L G A W V
HLH1 hu      W A P E Q P D DWYGHGLGGGE D C A H F - - - - - - T D D G A W N D D V C Q A P Y A W V
HL2a hu      W A V T Q P D NWHGHELGGSE D C V E V - - - - - - Q P D G A W N D D F C L Q V Y A W V
HL2 ra       W A F T Q P D NCQGHEEGGSE D C A E I - - - - - - L S D G L W N D N F C Q Q V N A W A
HL2a ra      W A F T Q P D NCQGHEEGGSE D C A E I - - - - - - L S D G L W N N D F C Q Q V N A W A
HL ch        W K E G E P N N A G F N E D C A H V - - - - - - W T S G Q W N D V Y C T Y E C Y Y V
CsPCP        W A P N Q P D N F F A TGE D C V VMI W - - - - - H E A G E W N D V P C N Y Q L P F T
PCP ch       W A P N Q P D NFF F A G E D C V VMI W - - - - - H E Q G E W N D V P C N Y H L P F T
LFIFI        W S E N N P D N Y K H Q E H C V H I W D T - - K P L Y Q W N D N D C N V K M G Y I
LECab        W S S N N P N N W E N - Q D C G V V N Y D - - T V T G Q W D D D D C N K N K N F L
MBPC ra      W N E G E P N N V G S G E N C V V L - - - - - - L T N G K W N D V P C S D S F L V V
```

FIGURE 1

Alignment of the carboxyterminal portion of the animal lectin domain of mLHR (amino acids 76-118) and comparison to the similar region in other proteins containing this motif. The relative enrichment in lysines in this region is emphasized.

and no Lys (Fig. 1). Other mammalian lectins containing Lys in this region are the mannose binding protein-C (MBP-C) of rat and human, and human IgE Fc receptor, each of which has a single Lys, and canine pulmonary surfactant a with 2 Lys. Because MEL-14, a functional epitope, appears to recognize a ubiquitin-dependent determinant, the striking preponderance of Lys in the region suggests possible candidate sites for ubiquitination. Alternatively, of course, this may reflect a requirement for interaction with an anionic carbohydrate moiety, a carbohydrate requirement that has been delineated (Yednock and Rosen, 1989).

We have also studied the progression of events in the biosynthesis of $gp90^{MEL\text{-}14}$ in an effort to explain the difference in molecular weight between the core protein of 37 kD and the 95 kD mature molecule (Van de Rijn *et al.*, 1990). Pulse labeling experiments showed a rapid synthesis of a 70 kD precursor form containing high mannose, N-linked oligosaccharides. On processing of the high mannose oligosaccharides into complex N-linked oligosaccharides, the precursor matures in a single step into the 95 kD form. Experiments using deglycosylating enzymes and inhibitors of N-linked glycosylation demonstrated that the molecular weight of deglycosylated $gp90^{MEL\text{-}14}$ is 45 kD and that processing to the mature 95 kD form from the 45 kD form results from extensive N-linked glycosylation. The core protein molecular weight of *in vitro* transcribed and translated $gp90^{MEL\text{-}14}$ cDNA is consistent with the estimated molecular weight of 37 kD, predicted from the cDNA sequence of the core protein, and 8 to 10 kD less than the molecular weight of deglycosylated $gp90^{MEL\text{-}14}$ produced in cells in the presence of tunicamycin (45 kD). Because glycosylation cannot account for this discrepancy, this adds further evidence that addition of one ubiquitin moiety to the core protein during biosynthesis occurs.

III. Structural Analysis of Lymph Node Homing Receptor cDNA

The three cell surface glycoproteins comprising this new family of adhesion molecules are all transmembrane proteins with an unusual protein mosaic architecture. They each contain a tandem array of three kinds of domains: a calcium dependent animal lectin domain, an EGF-like domain, and a variable number of repeat units, conforming to the short consensus repeats of complement regulatory and other proteins (Bevilacqua *et al.*, 1989; Johnston *et al.*, 1989; Lasky *et al.*, 1989; Siegelman *et al.*, 1989) (Fig. 2). The peripheral lymph node homing receptor member LHR ($gp90^{MEL\text{-}14}$, LAM-1) is present on lymphocytes and mediates the adherence of lym-

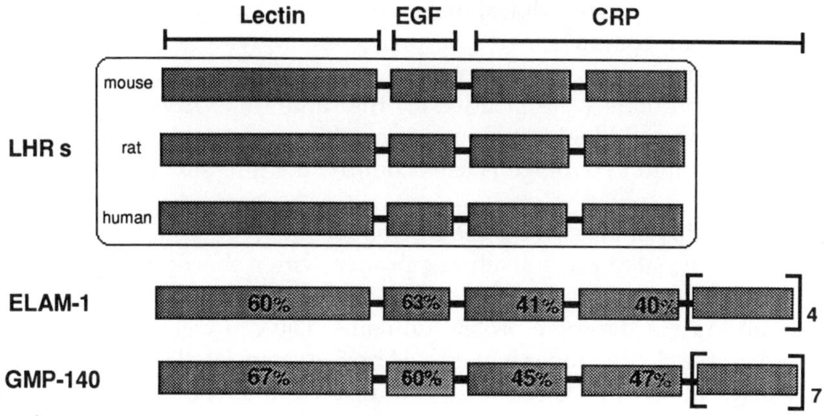

FIGURE 2

Comparison of the SELECTIN family of adhesion molecules. The lymph node homing receptor is compared to the other two members of the family, ELAM-1 and GMP-140. Percentages refer to protein sequence identity in each domain compared to that of mouse LHR.

phocytes to endothelial cells of high endothelial venules in peripheral lymph nodes (Gallatin *et al.*, 1983) and on neutrophils similarly involved in their extravasation at inflammatory sites (Lewinsohn *et al.*, 1987). Endothelial leukocyte adhesion molecule-1 (ELAM-1) is a cell surface structure expressed on cytokine induced endothelial cells (Bevilacqua *et al.*, 1987) and mediates the binding of leukocytes. GMP-140 (PADGEM, CD62) is contained and stored within alpha granules of platelets and Weibel–Palade bodies of endothelial cells (Hsu-Lin *et al.*, 1984; McEver and Martin, 1984), is rapidly mobilized to the cell surface on activation, and promotes binding of these cells to monocytes and neutrophils (Hamburger and McEver, 1990; Larsen *et al.*, 1989).

The analysis of aminoterminal amino acid sequence of the core polypeptide of the mouse lymph node homing receptor (mLHRc) lead to preparation of an oligonucleotide probe that allowed isolation and characterization of a cDNA clone encoding the core polypeptide of gp90MEL-14 (Siegelman *et al.*, 1989). The distribution of expression of the hybridizing transcripts to this cDNA was largely restricted to hematolymphoid cells and tissues. All cell lines and tissues expressing detectable mRNA, except testis, exhibited identical patterns with bands at 1.5, 2.5, and 5.2 kb. Expression of the transcript in northern blots from MEL-14 based cell line variants showed cosegregation of transcript and cell–surface antigen expression; therefore, qualitative and quantitative cell surface expression paralleled closely transcript abundance in these murine lymphoma cell lines. Normal tissues showed a predominant lymphoid distribution, paralleling tissue staining patterns for MEL-14. Thymus, spleen, and mesenteric lymph node were positive for the same transcripts found in cell lines, while liver, kidney, and brain showed no appreciable hybridization. Transfection into heterologous cells confirmed expression of the MEL-14 epitope.

Examination of the mLHRc cDNA clone sequence revealed a potentially highly glycosylated transmembrane protein with a short cytoplasmic tail. Unusual features inherent in the sequence include an extracytoplasmic tandem array of the three protein domains. The complete nucleotide sequence of the cDNA clone showed a 54 bp 5′ untranslated region followed by a single initiator ATG codon, beginning an uninterrupted open reading frame of 1116 bp. The TGA stop codon at position 1170 is followed by 327 bp of 3′ untranslated region in the mouse. The assignment of the initiator ATG is supported by the presence of a flanking sequence falling within those typifying eukaryotic initiator sites, in this case GCCATGG (Kozak, 1984).

The reading frame encodes a protein with a partite hydrophilic hydrophobic leader sequence 38 amino acids in length, before the initial tryptophan residue of the mature protein. The length of the leader sequence is unusual for a eukaryotic signal sequence. While hydropathy analysis (Kyte and Doolittle, 1982) confirms a generally hydrophobic leader sequence, the initial 15 residues are neutral to slightly hydrophilic. The apparent signal sequence is also distinctive in that it is enriched in cysteine (4 residues) and histidine (3 residues), largely clustered in the 12 residues preceding the mature protein. The combined unusual features suggest the possibility of specialized pathways of intracellular traffic.

The mature protein begins with a tryptophan, a highly unusual aminoterminal amino acid. Database searches reveal less than 10 sequences containing tryptophan as an aminoterminal residue. Three of these are peptide hormones, generally generated by cleavage of longer polypeptide chains. Only one of the remaining is a eukaryotic sequence. In this regard it should be noted that all three members of the SELECTIN family as well as all three of the homing receptor molecules in different species we have thus far examined appear to initiate with tryptophan.

The clone possesses 10 potential asparagine-linked glycosylation sites, consistent with our protein characterization studies showing extensive glycosylation on endoglycosidase F digestion (Siegelman *et al.*, 1986; Van de Rijn *et al.*, 1990) and subsequent tunicamycin inhibition experiments (Van de Rijn *et al.*, 1990). Six of these are contained within the identical complement regulatory protein (CRP) repeat unit structure. No clusters of

Ser, Thr, or both, characteristic of sites of O-linked glycosylation, are present in the deduced sequence, an observation confirming our inability to find evidence for O-linked glycosylation in cell surface and metabolic labeling studies of gp90MEL-14 (Van de Rijn *et al.*, 1990). The mature protein contains 22 cysteine residues, comprising 6.6 mole percent. Twelve of the cysteines are present in the CRP repeat structures, and an additional nine cysteines are concentrated in the 60 amino acids just preceding the repeat units in the EGF domain and carboxyterminal lectin domain, resulting in a highly cysteine rich pretransmembrane region of 180 to 190 amino acids.

The deduced mature protein is 334 amino acids in length, with a calculated molecular weight of 37,600. An hydrophobic transmembrane region encompassing amino acids from about 295 to 317 is followed by a cluster of positively charged residues and a hydrophilic cytoplasmic tail of 18 amino acids. Hydropathy analysis further shows distinct regions of relative hydrophilicity concentrated in the aminoterminal (150 amino acids) and in the membrane proximal (20 amino acids). The intervening extracytoplasmic portion is composed of a relatively electrical neutral stretch that includes EGF and CRP domains.

One type of carbohydrate binding protein, calcium dependent (C-type) animal lectins, are generally homologous to each other in a carboxyterminal domain of 130 to 150 residues, a region containing the carbohydrate binding activity, most intensively and earliest studied in the asialoglycoprotein receptor (Chiacchia and Drickamer, 1984; Drickamer, 1989; Drickamer, *et al.*, 1984; Spiess and Lodish, 1985; Spiess *et al.*, 1985). The mLHRc contains a motif homologous to this type of lectin, in particular to the hepatic lectins of human and rat over the aminoterminal 118 amino acids, particularly preserved over a stretch of 45 amino acids (74 to 118) bearing similarity to the 50 carboxyterminal residues of the binding domain in animal lectins. This region includes three invariant cysteines at 90, 109, and 116 in mLHRc, Asn-Trp at 75 to 76, a characteristic Glu-Pro-Asn (80 to 82), a Glu88, Cys-Val at 90 to 91, and the conserved Gly---Trp-Asn-Asp at 102 to 106. Only a highly conserved Gly12 in the consensus sequence and present in other mammalian lectins is absent from the presumed carbohydrate binding domain in mLHRc. As mentioned, a relative enrichment in positively charged residues and particularly lysines in this domain may have implications for sites of ubiquitination, carbohydrate binding, or both. The orientation of the lectin domain in mLHRc (and in all of the SELECTIN molecules) is unusual, being inverted with respect to most other animal lectins that are oriented with the aminoterminus anchored in the membrane and the carboxyterminus containing the binding portion extracytoplasmically.

The presence of a lectin domain in gp90^{MEL-14} is entirely consistent with studies that have demonstrated that some carbohydrates, mannose-6-phosphate and some analogues, but not other carbohydrates, inhibit binding to peripheral lymph node HEV but not Peyer's patch (Stoolman and Rosen, 1983; Stoolman *et al.*, 1984; Yednock and Rosen, 1989). MEL-14 has also been shown to inhibit specifically the binding of lymphocytes to polystyrene beads derivatized with PPME (a phosphomonoester mannan fragment rich in mannose-6-phosphate), suggesting a close association of these determiniants; yet excess soluble PPME does not inhibit binding of MEL-14 to cells (Yednock *et al.*, 1987); therefore, identity of the MEL-14 and carbohydrate-binding determinants is unlikely. Because MEL-14 appears to recognize a ubiquitin dependent determinant (Siegelman *et al.*, 1986; St. John *et al.*, 1986), the striking preponderance of Lys in the region suggests possible candidate sites for ubiquitination.

The EGF-like domain in mLHRc consists of a single copy homologue of the EGF repeat unit, which preserves many of the Cys/Gly residues characteristic of this structure (118-155). All six consensus cysteines are present as well as Gly147 and Gly150, and Tyr148 of mLHRc. The relationship (alignment) of these conserved residues is identical to that of human and bovine blood clotting factors IX and X and the drosophila notch gene product (in all but 4 of 36 repeats in this gene) but not to the other molecules containing EGF-like domains. Moreover, the best fit with all of the EGF-like units examined was with repeats 26 and 14 of D. Notch, and it is similar to some other of the EGF units in the four neurogenic loci in *Drosophila melanogaster.* It is striking that these molecules, apparently mediating early cell–cell interaction events in embryogenesis controlling the developmental choice of ectodermal cells to either neural or epidermal pathways, provide some of the best alignments and similarities to the LHRs. In fact, D. Notch has been demonstrated to have a role in cell–cell interaction (Fehon *et al.*, 1990; Kidd *et al.*, 1986; Wharton *et al.*, 1985). It is also of special interest that this EGF-like domain shares homology with a portion of one of the cysteine rich repeat units of the beta chain of the integrin LFA-1 β2 chain in the human (positions 449 to 483). A 12 amino acid region comprising mLHRc 142 to 154 aligns directly with 480 to 482 of the LFA-1 β2 subunit, retaining the conserved spacing of three cysteines, with identity of seven residues (58%). With additional conserved amino acids included, 10 residues (83%) are homologous. While of uncertain significance over a short region, this relationship to integrins is of interest, with our laboratory's discovery that Peyer's patch homing is governed by an integrin with a previously uncharacterized β chain βp (Holzmann *et al.*, 1989; Holzmann and Weissman, 1989), and this chain indeed shows four cysteine rich repeats homologous to EGF domains (See Chapter 5).

The third homology domain preserves the protein motif of short consensus repeats seen in complement regulatory and other proteins. Each unit is 62 amino acids in length, spans positions 156 to 217 and 218 to 279, and is completely identical at the nucleotide as well as protein levels. The murine complement factor H, a serum protein with complement regulatory activity (Kristensen and Tack, 1986) was identified as homologous over this region in data bank searches using the protein search algorithm FASTP (Lipman and Pearson, 1985). In factor H, there are 20 contiguous homologous, though not identical, repeat units having approximately 10 to 31% homology with this domain of the mLHRc receptor. The same homologous repeat motif exists in a number of complement regulatory proteins that bind the cleaved forms of C3 and C4 (reviewed in Ahearn and Fearon, 1989; Hourcade *et al.*, 1989; Reid and Day, 1989) and in other proteins such as the Il-2 receptor (Ishida *et al.*, 1985; Leonard *et al.*, 1985), the β2-glycoprotein serum protein (Lozier *et al.*, 1984), and factor XIII (Ichinose *et al.*, 1986). Every consensus sequence position is represented in the homing receptor repeat unit sequence. Except for a relative deletion of one residue between Cys4 and Pro7 of the consensus sequence, and an insertion of three residues between Pro7 and Phe30, the relative spacing of the remaining residues of the consensus sequence is completely preserved in the homing receptor sequence. Two additional cysteines are also present in the homing receptor (and other SELECTIN molecules) repeats relative to all other such units. Comparison to the repeat units of noncomplement proteins Interleukin-2 receptor, beta2-glycoprotein I, and factor XII shows greater similarity of the homing receptor repeat structure to complement than to noncomplement proteins. While homologous repeat units are not unusual among cell surface and other proteins, the presence of a precisely identical repeat unit from nucleotide positions 633 to 818 and 819 to 1005 is distinctive, and is not preserved in man (Siegelman and Weissman, 1989) or rat (unpublished observations). The finding of an identical rather than homologous repeat of the CRP-like sequence is striking. This implies a very recent gene segment duplication, rather than a reduction to two units from a multiunit ancestor segment by unequal crossing over. It will be of interest to trace the evolutionary history of this unit in a more precise way.

IV. Evolutionary Conservation of Lymphocyte Homing Receptor Structure

In the human, a cell surface molecule, $gp90^{Hermes}$, had also been identified that structurally and functionally was thought to represent the human counterpart to $gp90^{MEL\text{-}14}$ (Jalkanen *et al.*, 1986) and in fact was reported to bear antigenic relationship to it (Jalkanen *et al.*, 1988). Molecular cloning in both the human and primate has shown this molecule to be equivalent to CD44, Pgp-1, and the ECMIII receptor (Goldstein *et al.*, 1989; St John *et al.*, 1990; Stamenkovic *et al.*, 1989) but is unrelated to the mLHR that encodes $gp90^{MEL-14}$. Similarly, characterization of lymph node and Peyer's patch homing receptors in the rat has lead to the description of a number of molecular species apparently disparate from those of mouse (Chin *et al.*, 1986; Rasmussen *et al.*, 1985; Woodruff *et al.*, 1987). In order to determine whether or not a homologous protein to the mLHRc is expressed in human and rat and to address evolutionary issues posed by the unusual mLHRc composition, we isolated the human and rat cDNAs encoding homologues to mLHRc (Fig. 3).

Because RNA blot analysis for the mouse homing receptor clone showed distribution of transcripts limited to lymphod tissues and lymphoma cell lines showing cell surface expression of $gp90^{MEL-14}$, an RNA blot was performed using RNA from a panel of normal human tissues and cell lines, and an isolated full length hLHRc clone as probe. A single predominant transcript of about 2.5 kb was identified in contrast to the pattern in the mouse (Siegelman *et al.*, 1989), in which two additional hybridizing species of 1.5 and 5.2 kb exist. Nonetheless, in precise analogy to the mouse, expression of transcripts was limited to blood and lymphoid tissues. PBL, tonsil, and thymus were positive, while detectable transcripts were absent from liver, brain, and placenta. It is of note that the thymus transcript is 200 to 300 bp larger than all other transcripts from tissues or cell lines. The transcript was identified also in lymphoid cell lines, and exclusively in those known to have peripheral node HEV binding activity. Therefore, in all tissues and cell lines examined the pattern of transcript

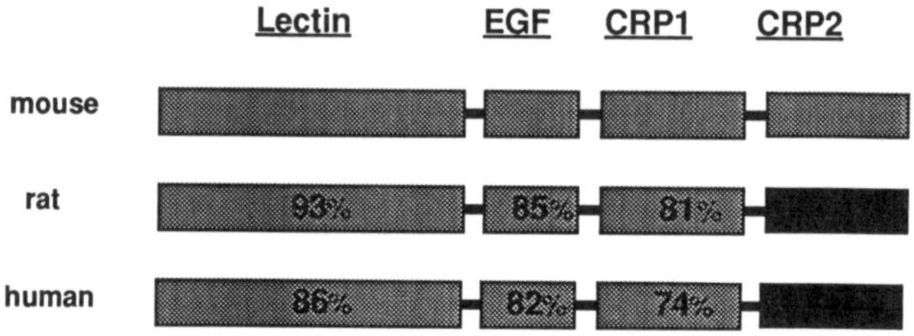

FIGURE 3

Cross-species comparison between mouse, man, and rat of the amino acid sequences of the three genre of protein domains in the lymph node homing receptor. Percentages refer to sequence identity in each domain to that of mouse LHRc.

expression parallels that seen in the mouse with restriction to hemato-lymphoid tissues and lymphoid cell lines that exhibit significant HEV binding capacity. This is in contrast to CD44 distribution, which has been shown to be expressed quite broadly in tissues and cell lines (Picker *et al.*, 1989) aparently independently of lymph node homing capacity. Because the MEL-14 epitope in the mouse is transiently expressed at high levels in the thymus during embryonic development at a stage when a subset of mature Tγ/δ cells (Vγ3, Vδ1) are poised to emigrate to the periphery and perhaps exclusively to the skin (Havran and Allison, 1988) and expression is restricted architecturally in the adult mouse thymus, the altered transcript size could have functional significance.

The initiator ATG in the 2,354 bp human clone is preceded by 115 bp of 5′ untranslated region and is followed by an uninterrupted reading frame of 1002 bp and 1123 bp of 3′ untranslated region succeeding the TAA stop codon. Identical to the mouse, the predicted protein, including signal sequence in man and rat, is also 374 amino acids long. The mature core protein is 334 amino acids with a predicted unmodified polypeptide size of 37,402 D. All three species contain 22 conserved cysteine residues with the relationships of all completely conserved. Nineteen of these are concentrated in the CRP and EGF-like domains. The overall identity of mouse and human sequences is 77% at the amino acid and 79% at the nucleotide levels. For the mature protein, there is 80% identity and 85% similarity when considering conservative substitutions. Mouse and rat sequences show 86% identity for the mature protein. Comparison for each of the domains is shown in Fig. 3.

Potential N-linked glycosylation sites number eight in the human, whereas ten have been identified in the mouse and seven in the rat. Five of these in the human sequence are identical in position to the mouse; in particular, both sites in the lectin domain and the single site in the EGF domain align. These three are also conserved in the rat. Mouse and rat also preserve two sites in the first complement regulatory repeat, and one in the second. As in the mouse, no Ser/Thr rich regions are present in human or rat clones to suggest the presence of O-linked glycosylation. The least conserved region with respect to potential glycosylation sites is localized to the carboxyterminal CRP homologous repeat.

The leader sequence of human and rat clones is 38 amino acids long and identical in length to the mouse; as we have noted (Siegelman *et al.*, 1989), this is unusually long for a eukaryotic secreted or cell surface protein. Outside of a short stretch of nine amino acids from -31 to -24, where the sequences diverge considerably, the leader sequences are quite conserved between man and mouse for this evolutionary distance. Over this region of disparity between man and mouse with 12% identity, the identity between rat and man is 62%, in contrast to the remainder of the molecule where the expected greater similarity between rat and mouse prevails. There is an overall 63% identity and 82% similarity when conserved substitutions are included. Among the conserved residues are the three cysteines and two of the three histidines of the mouse. These are all conserved in the rat. The peculiar features of this signal sequence do not appear to be requisite for this class of cell–surface adhesion molecules, because ELAM-1, an endothelial adhesion molecule, has a very similar structure (Bevilacqua *et al.*, 1989), yet its leader sequence has no significant homology to those of the LHRs. GMP-140 has a very long leader sequence (Johnston *et al.*, 1989), but the sequence is otherwise quite dissimilar from the LHRs' sequence. The degree of conservation of length and sequence between these LHRs in this region suggests possible stringent structural constraints for the function of this leader perhaps reflecting specialized pathways of intracellular traffic. The putative transmembrane region (296 to 317) shows complete identity between mouse and human forms with the exception of a single conservative Ile–Leu interchange at position 313. The rat is completely identical to mouse in this region. The eight residues preceding and the initial nine intracytoplasmic residues, with positively charged residues consistent with a stop transfer sequence, following the hydrophobic transmembrane region are also completely conserved resulting in a 39 amino acid stretch of virtual identity, the longest region of identity among the molecules. In all three species the carboxyterminus of the molecule ends with a Tyr, an amino acid implicated in recognition events initiating internalization into clathrin coated pits (Pearse, 1988). This may have implications for some biosynthetic properties of $gp90^{MEL\text{-}14}$.

It is clear that the variety, number, and relationship of extracytoplasmic domains in the homing receptor cDNAs are preserved among the three species we have examined. The lectin family of proteins have demonstrated a common structural basis (Chiacchia and Drickamer, 1984; Drickamer, 1989; Drickamer *et al.*, 1984; Spiess and Lodish, 1985; Spiess *et al.*, 1985). The animal lectin domain identified structurally in mLHRc has been shown to have a functional correlate, in that $gp90^{MEL\text{-}14}$ has been inferred to have lectin properties (Yednock and Rosen, 1989). These properties have been shown to extend to man and rat as well (Stoolman *et al.*, 1987). Human and mouse sequences shown 86% identity over this entire region, whereas rat and mouse show 93% identity with only a single difference in the carboxyterminal half (Fig. 3). Focally there are concentrated stretches of greater similarity between man and mouse, residues 1 to 12 (100% identity), 22 to 43 (95%), 48 to 97 (94%), and 102 to 120 (95%), regions that show increased conservation with ELAM-1 and GMP-140 as well. ELAM-1 in the same region is 59% identical to the human and 60% identical to the mouse LHRc. GMP-140 shows 65% identity to both human and mouse LHRs in this domain (Fig. 2). In addition, the ELAM-1 and GMP-40 sequences, unlike all the other animal lectins compared, requires no insertions or deletions for alignment with human or mouse LHRc sequences. Comparisons to the animal lectins most similar to thLHRc show the human lgE receptor and the human hepatic lectins having 32 and 28% identity, respectively. Earlier we had suggested that a relative lysine rich region in the LHRc lectin domain may provide clues to possible sites of ubiquitination. All of the seven Lys residues in this region in the mouse are precisely preserved in the human. All Lys in the lectin domain are conserved between mouse and rat. An additional eighth Lys is present in the human at position 99. Remarkably, ELAM-1 is also relatively Lys rich in this region with seven, including a cluster of three at 111 to 113. However, these are generally not ones shared identically with LHRs.

The second protein motif comprising residues 122 to 154 is related to proteins containing the EGF-like sequence (Cooke *et al.*, 1987). The human and mouse LHR sequences share 82% identity in this region, while the rat and mouse sequences are 85% similar (Fig. 3). In contrast to the lectin domain, comparisons of the corresponding EGF-like region of ELAM-1 to hLHRc shows somewhat greater similarity to the human sequence than the mouse, with 73 and 60% identity, respectively. GMP-140 shows about 60% identity to hLHRc in this region. Unlike the lectin domain, although human and mouse LHRs are more related to each other overall, the human sequences ELAM-1 and hLHRc show more similarity in the EGF-like domain than ELAM-1 to mLHRc. Within this domain, there is a 17 amino acid stretch of 100% identity (126 to 142) between hLHRc and ELAM-1, which is 82% conserved between mLHRc and both human proteins, perhaps suggesting possible common species specific structural requirements for function in this domain. For example, it is thought that the EGF domain in the LDL receptor is essential for recycling of the receptor back to the surface after endocytosis in clathrin coated pits (Davis *et al.*, 1987). Alternatively, the EGF domain in LHRs may subserve a separate protein–protein, cell–cell, or cell–matrix interactive role in the process of adhesion to HEVs or translocation through the vessel wall into lymph node (See following discussion). As mentioned four neurogenic loci in *Drosophila melanogaster* provide some of the best alignments and similarities to the LHRs.

CRPs generally share the property of binding to C3b and C4b of the complement cascade (reviewed in [Ahearn and Fearon, 1989; Hourcade *et al.*, 1989; Reid and Day, 1989]), thereby dampening the cascade at key amplification junctures, perhaps to protect host cells from complement lysis. Proteins apparently unrelated to this system also contain this motif, including the interleukin-2 receptor (Ishida *et al.*, 1985; Leonard *et al.*, 1985) and a human serum protein beta$_2$ glycoprotein I (Lozier *et al.*, 1984). In contrast to the mouse, the rLHR and hLHR CRP domains (155 to 278) each consist of two homologous (not identical) repeat units of 63 amino acids each. The human and rat CRP_1 and CRP_2 are quite divergent, sharing only about 60% of positions. However, both do retain the six cysteine pattern in both repeats, in common with ELAM-1 and GMP-140, but distinct from other CRP subunits that contain four. Comparisons between human and mouse LHRs show 74% conservation to CRP_1 and only 60% to CRP_2. If the more conserved aminoterminal 38 amino acids are considered alone, the mouse sequence shows 86% identity to CRP_1 and 67% to CRP_2. This suggests possible duplication of an ancestral segment related to the mouse CRP sequence—with relative preservation of this sequence in CRP_1 of the human and rat, particularly aminoterminally—and relative drift of the CRP_2 subunit. An alternative explanation of the identical repeats in the mouse is that there was an early domain duplication with a recent gene conversion event in the mouse resulting in the identical repeat. Examination of this receptor in wild mice and other murine subspecies should help distinguish the mechanism through which this arose. In any case, there appears to be a strict requirement for two CRP subunits in the LHRs, in contrast to the other SELECTINs. Alignment of the first CRP unit of ELAM-1 with CRP_1 and CRP_2 of hLHRc shows 41 and 40% identity, respectively. While less similar to the LHRs than in the lectin and EGF domains, the ELAM-1 CRP sequence is nonetheless more related to the LHRs than the most related other proteins in this region, with human complement factor H showing 35% and beta2 glycoprotein I showing 27% identity. It is attractive to consider that the CRP segment in LHRs has a complement regulatory function, which might seem an appropriate role for structures on cells recruited to and at inflammatory sites [i.e., lymphocytes (LHRs) and activated endothelial cells (ELAM-1 and GMP-140)]. Indeed, the MEL-14 epitope has also been identified on mouse neutrophils and is thought to be implicated in participating in extravasation of these cells at inflammatory sites (Lewinsohn *et al.*, 1987).

The high degree of structural conservation with a molecule known to confer specific lymphocyte homing activity in another species, and the restricted lymphoid expression of transcript, in strict analogy to the mouse, strongly suggested that a cell surface molecule most likely mediates a similar function in the human. We have transfected both mouse and human cDNAs into a mouse lymphoid cell line with no known HEV-binding specificity and have obtained stable high level surface expression. Application of these cells in both *in vitro* and *in vivo* homing assays demonstrated the expected functional HEV binding (unpublished observations). It is yet to be determined whether the structurally highly homologous rat LHR will also fulfill these expectations.

A purported tissue specific lymphocyte-HEV adhesion system in the human has been described that also involves a cell surface gp90 species, designated $gp90^{Hermes}$ (Jalkanen *et al.*, 1986). The molecule is sulfated and modified by O-linked as well as N-linked glycosylation (Jalkanen *et al.*, 1988) in contrast to $gp90^{MEL\text{-}14}$, which we have shown to contain glycosylation only in N-linked form (Van de Rijn *et al.*, 1990). Expression of $gp90^{Hermes}$ is not restricted to hematolymphoid cell types (Picker *et al.*, 1989). However, the $gp90^{Hermes}$ molecule in humans apparently participates in specific binding by direct evidence to mucosal sites and is claimed, by indirect evidence, also to be responsible for binding to peripheral lymph node sites. In contrast, as mentioned, specific binding of human and mouse lymphocytes to mucosal site HEVs in the mouse utilizes an α/βintegrin heterodimer related to VLA-4 (Holzmann *et al.*, 1989); there is not yet a known requirement for or participation of any gp90 species in Peyer's patch binding in the mouse. Molecular cloning of $gp90^{Hermes}$ (Goldstein *et al.*, 1989; Stamenkovic *et al.*, 1989) and its counterpart in the primate $gp90^{Hutch}$ (St John *et al.*, 1990) reveal identity to previously described molecules with a wide distribution, CD44, Pgp-1, and the ECMIII receptor (Carter and Wayner, 1988; Dalchau *et al.*, 1980; Trowbridge, *et al.*, 1982). The cloned molecule is related to regions of the cartilage proteoglycan core and link proteins. It contains no sequences related to any of the three major homologous domains of human and mouse LHRcs, and shows no significant sequence homology to hLHRc. It has also been reported that the monoclonal antibody MEL-14, used to define peripheral lymph node homing in the mouse (Gallatin *et al.*, 1983) can block adhesion of human lymphocytes to HEV *in vitro* and that it has been reported that $gp90^{Hermes}$- bears the MEL-14 epitope (Jalkanen *et al.*, 1988). Because the primary structure of $gp90^{Hermes}$ and hLHRc are so disparate, it is unclear whether or not this represents commonality of some post-transcriptional modification such as ubiquitination, fortuitous cross-reaction, or otherwise artifactual. It is unlikely that mice and humans utilize completely different systems governing lymphocyte-HEV adhesion, because the adhesive event is preserved across these species (Butcher and Weissman, 1980). Indeed, transfection and stable expression of hLHRc cDNA in lymphoid cells shows the expected peripheral lymph node HEV binding (unpublished observations). It is possible that both $gp90^{Hermes}$ and hLHRc act in conjunction as a receptor complex. However, this suggestion conflicts with our observations in the mouse, which have shown frequent completely discordant expression of gp90$^{MEL\text{-}14}$ and Pgp-1 (in preparation).

V. Conservation of a Chromosomal Region Containing the Lymph Node Homing Receptor, Its Gene Family, and Complement Regulatory Genes

We have described chromosomal mapping of mLHRc to distal chromosome 1, inseparable in recombinant inbred strains from the lymphocyte surface marker Ly-22 (Siegelman *et al.,* 1990; Watson *et al.,* 1990). The human homologue (hLHRc, LAM-1) has also been localized to chromosome 1 (Tedder *et al.,* 1989). We have confirmed this mapping by other techniques for hLHRc, as well as by interspecific crosses for mLHRc (Watson *et al.,* 1990), and have demonstrated coclustering of the two other proteins with a similar tridomain protein architecture on a distal segment of chromosome 1 in the mouse syntenic with human chromosome 1q (Watson *et al.,* 1990): Thus, it is clear that structural similarity has correctly predicted a new gene family of tridomain chimeric protein adhesion molecules. The syntenic portion of chromosome 1 between man and mouse is known to house many characterized complement binding and complement regulatory protein genes (Ahearn and Fearon, 1989; Hourcade *et al.,* 1989; Reid and Day, 1989). This family is characterized structurally by the conserved 62 amino acid repeat motif (short consensus repeats) shared with the two extracytoplasmic carboxyterminal domains of the lymph node homing receptor. Indeed, the major difference among these three members is the variable number of CRP units they contain; LHRs of human, mouse, and rat containing two, ELAM-1 with six, and GMP-140 with nine. It therefore appears that it is the sequences within the CRP units that have served as the dominant or perhaps primordial sequences determining colocalization on chromosome 1. Closer examination of this region will be of particular interest to address whether or not driving forces other than recent duplication have contributed to the clustering and high degree of relatedness of these receptor molecules. Because SELECTINs have thus far been detected on the two cellular participants in the extravasation of hematolymphoid cells, lymphocytes or neutrophils, and the endothelial cell, it is tempting to speculate that coordinate regulation of gene expression places evolutionary pressure maintaining their proximity.

It should be noted that maps of mouse chromosome 1 place Ly-22 centromeric to the antithrombin III (At-3) gene. This marker has served as an "anchor" locus in the mouse, defined by three-point crosses and extensive data (Seldin *et al.*, 1988a,b). Yet, fine RFLP mapping utilizing *mus spretus* backcross mice clearly places mLHRc telomeric to At-3 (Watson *et al.*, 1990). If true, this would imply separate loci for these, contrary to evidence that supports the identity of mLHR and Ly-22. The apparent discrepancy can be explained easily by examination of the original criteria for placing Ly-22 centromeric to At-3. In fact, only a single crossover event in recombinant inbred mice separated At-3 and Ly-22, and therefore, the crossover frequency gave an appropriate distance but the placement on either side of At-3 was arbitrary (Ben Taylor, Jackson Laboratory, personal communication). Given our unambiguous positioning of mLHRc telomeric to At-3 in *mus spretus* backcross mice by RFLP mapping (Watson *et al.*, 1990), we conclude that Ly-22 is properly placed at about the same distance from but telomeric to At-3 and that the mouse chromosome 1 map requires an ammendment to reflect this.

VI. Functional Domains of the Lymph Node Homing Receptor

Well before the elucidation of the structure of SELECTIN proteins, evidence for a carbohydrate component in the high endothelial ligand for the $gp90^{MEL-14}$ molecule existed. *In vitro* homing receptor activity could be abrogated specifically by the monosaccharides mannose-6-phosphate and the structurally related fructose-1-phosphate. In addition, two polysaccharides, fucoidin and PPME, the latter a yeast derivative core mannan rich in mannose-6-phosphate, were found to be potent inhibitors of binding as well reviewed in Yednock and Rosen, (1989). It has been further demonstrated that sialidase treatment of HEV ablates binding of both lymphocytes and recombinant $gp90^{MEL-14}$ to tissue sections and the *in vivo* binding of lymphocytes to HEV (Yednock and Rosen, 1989), confirming the anionic requirement for the carbohydrate based portion of the binding. Because discrete forms of sialic acid form the basis of influenze virus binding to erythrocytes (Paulson, 1985; Wiley and Skehel, 1987) and extensive information can potentially be contained in the diversity of sialidation events, it is attractive to suggest that a form of sialic acid contributes to the recognition structure itself. These studies have contributed greatly to our understanding of the lectin nature of the LHR SELECTIN, but the actual physiological ligand on the high endothelial cell has remained elusive. Investigations have directly addressed the carboydrate ligand for ELAM-1 and GMP-140 (Goelz *et al.*, 1990; Larsen *et al.*, 1990; Lowe *et al.*, 1990; Phillips *et al.*, 1990; Tiemeyer *et al.*, 1991; Walz *et al.*, 1990).

Although these studies characterize the specific form of lectin based carbohydrate binding to the human blood group antigen Lewis X (GMP-140) or sialyl Lewis X (ELAM-1), major issues still remain. The minimal carbohydrate structures identified only begin the search for the actual physiological ligands. There is also no complete assurance that these carbohydrate inhibitors represent the precise structures on the cells bearing the complementary ligand. For instance, lacto-N-fucopentaose III (LNFIII), or Lewis X, is only inhibitory of GMP-140 binding at relatively high concentrations and is maximally only 70 to 80% complete (Larsen *et al.*, 1990). Moreover, the closely related LNFII also shows some inhibition. The ELAM-1 specificity for sialylated Lewis X, SLe^x is perhaps more complete in all of these studies, but a well-characterized closely related derivative, a difucosylated form, is completely inhibitory (Phillips *et al.*, 1990). It is clear that the *complete* carbohydrate structures of the ligands must still be elucidated, and the identities of the protein or lipid molecules bearing these carbohydrates are as yet unknown. Although patterns of glycosylation are determined broadly for a cell type, perhaps only one or a few of the properly glycosylated cell surface species are relevant to functional adherence, subsequent signaling or translocation (transendothelial migration), or both events.

Though it is clear that the aminoterminal lectin domain clearly plays a crucial role in the adhesive function of these receptors, it is best to acknowledge the high degree of structural conservation among the other two domain motifs across species for LHR (Bowen *et al.*, 1980; Siegelman and Weissman, 1989; Tedder *et al.*, 1989) and among members of the family. In fact, conservation of amino acid sequence in the EGF-like domain is equivalent to that of the lectin domains (Fig. 3). It should be noted that there may be some dependence of expression of lectin determinants on the presence of the EGF domain (Walz *et al.*, 1990). However, our evidence indicates that the EGF domain of mLHR may contribute to HEV binding or events distal to the initial binding, and this may be independent of the receptor's lectin activity (Siegelman *et al.*, 1990). We demonstrated that the homing receptor locus is inseparable in recombinant inbred mouse strains from the polymorphic murine lymphocyte cell surface marker Ly-22. This marker is defined by a monoclonal antibody derived by alloimmunization of DBA/2 mice with a BALB/c neoplastic T-cell line (Tada *et al.*, 1983). The antibody was shown to identify the majority of lymph node cells and 30% of spleen cells, and to be present at lower levels in a number of other lymphoid but not nonlymphoid tissues. Staining of numerous cell lines and sources revealed identical staining patterns with Ly-22 and MEL-14. Immunoprecipitation further showed identically sized species on SDS gels under reducing and nonreducing conditions and transfection of mLHRc into eukaryotic cells resulted in expression of Ly-22. Together, these data indicated that Ly-22 is an allelic determinant on the lymph node homing receptor protein.

Because MEL-14 is a strong inhibitor of functional binding in the HEV assay (Gallatin *et al.*, 1983), appears to recognize a novel epitope on the homing receptor molecule composed of a combinatorial determinant between ubiquitin and the core polypeptide (Siegelman *et al.*, 1986; St John *et al.*, 1986), and has been associated with the carbohydrate-binding domain of the molecule (Yednock *et al.*, 1987), it was of interest to determine the relationship between Ly-22 and MEL-14 determinants. The results of antibody crossblocking studies demonstrated that while preincubation of cells with MEL-14 antibody does inhibit staining by MEL-14, preincubation with excess anti-Ly-22 has no effect on subsequent MEL-14 staining. This indicated that separate epitopes on the lymphocyte homing receptor are recognized by MEL-14 and anti-Ly-22 antibodies. It has been further shown that MEL-14 inhibits binding of PPME (a phosphomonoester mannan fragment rich in mannose-6-phosphate), a polysaccharide identifying the lectin activity of the peripheral node homing receptor (Yednock *et al.*, 1987a,b) to lymphocytes. We confirmed the expected inhibition of binding of fluoresceinated PPME to EL-$4^{MEL\text{-}14hi}$ cells pretreated with saturating levels of MEL-14. In contrast, preincubation with excess anti-Ly-22 had no detectable effect on subsequent staining with PPME. The level of staining seen after anti-Ly-22 is comparable to or actually enhanced over that seen with PPME alone or with preincubation with control antibodies. It was, therefore, clear by this independent criterion that the Ly-22 epitope is distinct from both MEL-14 and the lectin activity of the homing receptor.

We reported the sequence of an mLHR derived from an Ly-22^+ source EL-$4^{MEL\text{-}14hi}$ (Siegelman *et al.*, 1989) shown to be completely identical to the same molecule isolated from splenocytes from ICR mice (Lasky *et al.*, 1989). We, therefore, cloned the cDNA from an Ly-22^- strain, SJL, to determine the primary structural difference responsible for the antigenic polymorphism. The complete nucleotide sequence and protein translation of the Ly-22^- homing receptor sequence was compared to that of C3H/HEN (Ly-22^+) identically cloned and sequenced. The latter is completely identical to the previously reported mLHRc sequences (Lasky *et al.*, 1989; Siegelman *et al.*, 1989).

In the entire sequence of the Ly-22^- molecule, a total of four nucleotides differed. The only productive substitution within the entire coding portion of the mature polypeptide was the A-C interchange at nucleotide 604, resulting in a Glu (Ly-22$^-$) replacement of Ala (Ly-22$^+$) at amino acid 146. This site is in the carboxyterminal 10 amino acids of the EGF-like domain. As this single amino acid substitution, resulting in a charge difference, is the only primary structural difference in the mature protein between Ly-22$^+$ and Ly-22$^-$ mLHR molecules, this suggests that this difference likely forms the basis for the structural polymorphism giving rise to the Ly-22 epitope.

Until these studies, a single monoclonal Ab, MEL-14, has been available to define the mouse lymph node specific homing receptor. Moreover, the MEL-14 antigen has been shown to bear a relationship to the carbohydrate binding and functional portion of the molecule (Stoolman *et al.*, 1984; Yednock *et al.*, 1987a,b) and apparently resides in the lectin domain (Bowen *et al.*, 1990). This body of evidence strongly implicates the CHO binding lectin domain, containing the MEL-14 determinant, in adhesion to HEV. In order to determine whether or not anti-Ly-22 had any effect on the binding of lymphocytes to lymph node high endothelial venules, we applied the antibody in a modified Stamper and Woodruff *in vitro* HEV assay. The results demonstrated high efficiency blocking of peripheral node lymphocytes to lymph node high endothelial venules. Moreover, the extent of inhibition appeared at least comparable to that of MEL-14 under the same conditions. It appears, therefore, that a monoclonal antibody directed against the EGF domain of the lymph node homing receptor impedes binding of lymphocytes to HEV with high efficiency.

In summary, anti-Ly-22 defines a new functional and polymorphic determinant on gp90$^{MEL\text{-}14}$, and by primary structural analysis, localizes the Ly-22 epitope to the distal portion of the EGF domain. The functional aspect can be subjected to a number of interpretations. It is conceivable that a conformational change at a distance from the primary structural polymorphism in the lectin domain is recognized by anti-Ly-22. If so, from our evidence this disturbs neither carbohydrate nor MEL-14 binding. It is also clear that a Glu-Ala interchange, a net single negative charge difference, is sufficient to form the structural basis of the Ly-22 antigen. Moreover, the Glu-Ala interchange occurs at a residue that, in homologous domains in other proteins, allows considerable variation. Nine different residues in 21 different proteins, including Glu, are found at this position. All of the variants have a neutral or acid residue, inferring some constraint in the possibilities. Therefore, while we expect this change could form the basis of an antigenic determinant, we regard as unlikely that the overall conformation and disulfide structure of the domain is significantly disrupted by this. Thus, we conclude that unlike the complex epitope recognized by MEL-14, anti-Ly-22 recognizes a core polypeptide determinant. It nonetheless cannot be formally excluded that the anti-Ly-22 inhibition of HEV binding is due to secondary changes or steric influences induced, for example, in the lectin domain, where adhesive function has been expected to reside. However, we showed that anti-Ly-22 does not detectably impair carbohydrate binding activity. The most direct interpretation for the data, therefore, suggests the primary difference in the EGF-like domain is recognized, and this domain itself participates in the adhesion event, serving as at least part of the ligand for the peripheral node "addressin" molecules on the endothelial cell (Fig. 4). Examples of a direct role of an EGF moiety in protein–protein interactions exist. A portion of the EGF-like repeat domain of thrombomodulin, an endothelial cell surface glycoprotein, has been shown to act as the primary thrombin binding site (Kurosawa *et al.*, 1988). The EGF-like domain of plasminogen activator has also been shown to be the receptor binding portion (Appella and Blasi, 1987; Appella *et al.*, 1987). A precedent for a role for EGF domains in cell–cell interaction during embryogenesis in *Drosophila notch* protein, the EGF units of which bear some of the closest similarities to the EGF domain of the LHRs, has been delineated (Fehon *et al.*, 1990). A role for the EGF domain in HEV adhesion raises the speculative possibility that an EGF-like receptor serves as a ligand for LHR either as part of or in conjunction with the HEV addressin.

It should be noted that the standard frozen section HEV assay is likely a measure not only of the initial lumenal adhesive event of lymphocytes to high endothelial cells (HECs), but possibly of additional steps in the homing process before entry into lymph node parenchyma proper occurs. We have little knowledge of the events following initial adhesion at the lumenal surface or what other molecules may be involved, but vectorial translocation between or through layers of high-walled endothelium and then basement membrane must clearly ensue. In the frozen section assay, it is much more common to visualize oblique cross-sections of HEVs. The preponderance of binding that one measures may, therefore, be to endothelium below the lumenal surface, and it is conceivable that, because more than one event may be detected, inhibition of separate but necessary events in homing could be reflected by blocking by virtue of EGF or lectin domains. Alternatively, of course, there may simply be a requirement for at least two domains, EGF and lectin, to contribute to the initial adhesion with the addressin molecules (Fig. 4). The fact that both MEL-14 and anti-Ly-22 both block completely favors the interpretation that the functional regions defined by both antibodies largely overlap as to the steps in which these epitopes participate in the homing process. Beyond the functional roles of the other domains in the SELECTINs, questions of the subsequent signals transduced through these or associated molecules,

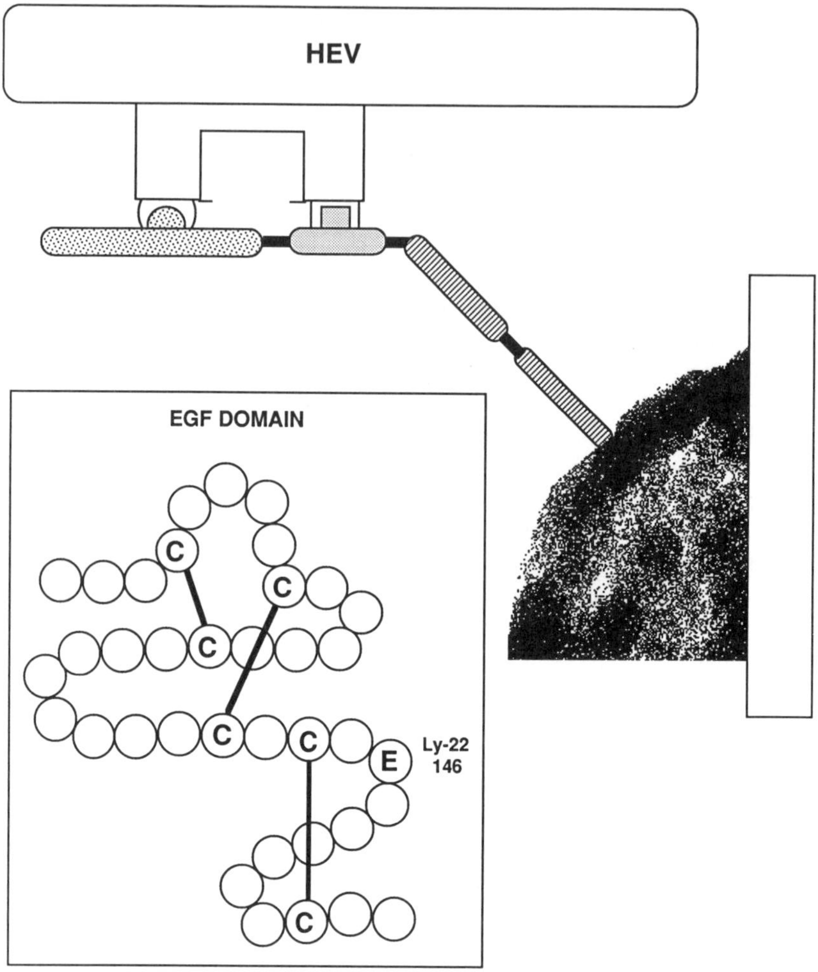

FIGURE 4

Schematic representation of the structures of lymph node homing receptors and their addressin ligand(s) on the high endothelial cell. Both lectin and EGF-like domains are hypothetically shown to interact with the complementary ligand on the endothelial cell. Inset shows the mLHR EGF-like domain modeled after the proposed three-dimensional structure of EGF (Cooke, 1987 #221). Structural localization of the polymorphic Ly-22 epitope to the glutamic acid at residue 146 is indicated.

their ligands, or both on either of the two participating cells, and the requirements for transendothelial migration provide ample territory to explore in the future.

VII. Broader Implications of the Lymph Node Homing Receptor for the Function of the Immune System

In studies using a number of leukocyte surface markers to identify T-cell functional subsets, Ly-22 was concluded to distinguish ConA-induced nonspecific T suppressor cells, positive for Ly-22, from helper and cytotoxic T-cells ($Ly\text{-}22^-$) (Chan *et al.*, 1983). Our understanding of LHR expression is that it is present during certain maturational stages of B- as well as T-cells, and that activation, at least to end stage differentiation, results in down regulation of the receptor in plasma cells and cytotoxic effector cells (Dailey *et al.*, 1985; Fink *et al.*, 1985; Reichert *et al.*, 1984; Reichert *et al.*, 1983; Reichert *et al.*, 1986) in general concordance with these observations, the human homologue of mLHRc, hLHRc (Siegelman and Weissman, 1989; Tedder *et al.*, 1989), which we have shown to confer functional HEV binding in transfected cells (in preparation), has been shown to encode the Leu-8 antigen (Camerini *et al.*, 1989). This antigen has been reported to delineate a T-cell subset of $CD4^+$ suppressor inducer, but not helper inducer phenotype (Kansas *et al.*, 1985a,b) Leu-8 is also absent from mature activated CTL (Takada *et al.*, 1989) in analogy with characterization of MEL-14 and Ly-22 in the mouse. The significance of the association of LHR expression and negative regulatory cells of the immune system remains to be clarified. However, it is conceivable that a preponderance of lymphocytes in the blood stream, which must be available to lymph node sites, function to control the amplitude of the immune response at the primary site where amplification occurs.

In this context, it may be pertinent to note the high frequency of autoimmune phenomena in $Ly\text{-}22^-$ strains (e.g., SJL, SWR, and NZB) relative to $Ly22^+$ strains. Although we have no evidence addressing whether or not the Ly-22 phenotype determines any functional differences in lymphocyte homing, it is tempting to speculate that there is a functional lymphocyte homing variation that influences autoimmune predispositions. These same strains have also been shown to share common T-cell receptor V_α haplotyeps in a large panel of normal and autoimmune mouse strains (Singer *et al.*, 1988). In this regard, it is important to note that the lineages of the $Ly\text{-}22^-$ strains (SJL, SWR/J, NZB, and DBA/2) are essentially completely independent (Altman and Dittmer-Katz, 1979). This suggests the possibility of a convergence to the Ly-22$^-$ sequence based on functional evolutionary pressures. A more likely explanation is that these two alleles are the most common in the larger wild population of mice and have been isolated in inbred strains. Instances of haplotypes in inbred strains being reflected in wild mouse populations have been observed (Rice and O'Brien, 1980). Furthermore, we have made the observation that LHR is expressed at a high level on the abnormal CD4$^-$CD8$^-$ T-cells that populate lymph nodes and blood in the autoimmune C3H gld/gld mouse (Roths *et al.*, 1984), suggesting that dysregulation of homing receptor expression may be related to disease progression (Siegelman *et al.*, 1991). The fact that there is colocalization of the gld locus and SELECTIN genes to a discrete region of chromosome 1 is also provocative and may indicate that loci in this region have significant effects on the regulation, development, and maturation of T-cells and the immune system.

References

Ahearn, J., and Fearon, D. (1989). *In* "Advances in Immunology" (F. Dixon, ed.), p. 183. Academic Press, New York.

Appella, E., and Blasi, F. (1987). *Ann. N.Y. Acad. Sci.* **511,** 192–195.

Appella, E., Robinson, E. A., Ullrich, S. J., Stoppelli, M. P., Corti, A., Cassani, G., and Blasi, F. (1987). *J. Biol. Chem.* **262,** 4437–4440.

Bargatze, R. F., Wu, N. W., Weissman, I. L., and Butcher, E. C. (1987). *J. Exp. Med.* **166,** 1125–1131.

Bevilacqua, M. P., Pober, J. S., Mendrick, D. L., Cotran, R. S., and Gimbrone, M. A., Jr. (1987). *Proc. Natl. Acad. Sci. U.S.A.* **84,** 9238–9242.

Bevilacqua, M. P., Stengelin, S., Gimbrone, M. A., Jr., and Seed, B. (1989). *Science* **243,** 1160–1165.

Bowen, B., Fennie, C., and Lasky, L. (1990). *J. Cell. Biol.* **110,** 147–153.

Bowen, B. R., Nguyen, T., and Lasky, L. A. (1989). *J. Cell. Biol.* **109,** 421–427.

Butcher, E. C., and Weissman, I. L. (1980). *Ciba. Found. Symp.*

Camerini, D., James, S. P., Stamenkovic, I., and Seed, B. (1989). *Nature (London)* **342,** 78–82.

Carter, W. G., and Wayner, E. A. (1988). *J. Biol. Chem.* **263,** 4193–4201.

Chan, M. M., Tada, N., Kimura, S., Hoffmann, M. K., Miller, R. A., Stutman, O., and Hammerling, U. (1983). *J. Immunol.* **130,** 2075–2078.

Chiacchia, K. B., and Drickamer, K. (1984). *J. Biol. Chem.* **259,** 15440–15446.

Chin, Y. H., Rasmussen, R. A., Woodruff, J. J., and Easton, T. G. (1986). *J. Immunol.* **136,** 2556–2561.

Cooke, R. M., Wilkinson, A. J., Baron, M., Pastore, A., Tappin, M. J., Campbell, I. D., Gregory, H., and Sheard, B. (1987). *Nature (London)* **327,** 339–341.

Dailey, M. O., Gallatin, W. M., and Weissman, I. L., (1985). *J. Mol. Cell. Immunol.* **2,** 27–36.

Dalchau, R., Kirkley, J., and Fabre, J. W. (1980). *Eur. J. Immunol.* **10,** 745–749.

Davis, C. G., Goldstein, J. L., Sudhof, T. C., Anderson, R. G., Russell, D. W., and Brown, M. S. (1987). *Nature (London)* **326,** 760–765.

Drickamer, K. (1989). *Biochem. Soc. Trans.* **17,** 13–15.

Drickamer, K., Mamon, J. F., Binns, G., and Leung, J. O. (1984). *J. Biol. Chem.* **259,** 770–778.

Fehon, R. G., Kooh, P. J., Rebay, I., Regan, C. L., Xu, T., Mushavitch, M. A., and Artavanis-Tsakonas, S. (1990). *Cell* **61,** 523–534.

Fink, P. J., Gallatin, W. M., Reichert, R. A., Butcher, E. C., and Weissman, I. L. (1985). *Nature (London)* **313,** 233–235.

Gallatin, W. M., Weissman, I. L., and Butcher, E. G. (1983). *Nature (London)* **304,** 30–34.

Goelz, S. E., Hession, C., Goff, D., Griffiths, B., Tizard, R., Newman, B., Chi-Rosso, G., and Lobb, R. (1990). *Cell* **63,** 1349–1356.

Goldstein, L. A., Zhou, D. F., Picker, L. J., Minty, C. N., Bargatze, R. F., Ding, J. F., and Butcher, E. C. (1989). *Cell* **56,** 1063–1072.

Gowans, J., and Knight, E. (1964). *Philos. Trans. R. Soc. (London)* **B 159,** 257–282.

Gutman, G., and Weissman, I. (1971). *Adv. Exp. Med. Biol.* **12,** 595–602.

Gutman, G. A., and Weissman, I. L. (1972). *Immunology* **23,** 465–479.

Gutman, G. A., and Weissman, I. L. (1973). *Transplantation* **16,** 621–629.

Hamburger, S. A., and McEver, R. P. (1990). *Blood* **75,** 550–554.

Havran, W. L., and Allison, J. P. (1988). *Nature (London)* **335,** 443–445.

Holzmann, B., McIntyre, B. W., and Weissman, I. L. (1989). *Cell* **56,** 37–46.

Holzmann, B., and Weissman, I. L. (1989). *Embo. J.* **8,** 1735–1741.

Hourcade, D., Holers, V. M., and Atkinson, J. P. (1989). *Adv. Immunol.*

Howard, J. C., Hunt, S. V., and Gowans, J. L. (1972). *J. Exp. Med.* **135,** 200–219.

Hsu-Lin, S., Berman, C. L., Furie, B. C., August, D., and Furie, B. (1984). *J. Biol. Chem.* **259,** 9121–9126.

Ichinose, A., McMullen, B. A., Fujikawa, K., and Davie, E. W. (1986). *Biochemistry* **25,** 4633–4638.

Idzerda, R. L., Carter, W. G., Nottenburg, C., Wayner, E. A., Gallatin, W. M., and St, John, T. (1989). *Proc. Natl. Acad. Sci. U.S.A.* **86,** 4659–4663.

Ishida, N., Kanamori, H., Noma, T., Nikaido, T., Sabe, H., Suzuki, N., Shimizu, A., and Honjo, T. (1985). *Nucleic Acids Res.* **13,** 7579–7589.

Jalkanen, S., Bargatze, R. F., de los Toyos, J., and Butcher, E. C. (1987). *J. Cell. Biol.* **105,** 983–990.

Jalkanen, S. T., Bargatze, R. F., Herron, L. R., and Butcher, E. C. (1986a). *Eur. J. Immunol.* **16,** 1195–1202.

Jalkanen, S., Jalkanen, M., Bargatze, R., Tammi, M., and Butcher, E. C. (1988). *J. Immunol.* **141,** 1615–1623.

Jalkanen, S., Reichert, R. A., Gallatin, W. M., Bargatze, R. F., Weissman, I. L., and Butcher, E. C. (1986b). *Immunol. Rev.* **91,** 39–60.

Johnston, G. I., Cook, R. G., and McEver, R. P. (1989). *Cell* **56,** 1033–1044.

Kansas, G. S., Wood, G. S., and Engleman, E. G. (1985a). *J. Immunol.* **134,** 3003–3006.

Kansas, G. S., Wood, G. S., Fishwild, D. M., and Engleman, E. G. (1985b). *J. Immunol.* **134,** 2995–3002.

Kidd, S., Kelley, M. R., and Young, M. W. (1986). *Mol. Cell. Biol.* **6,** 3094–3108.

Kozak, M. (1984). *Nucleic Acids Res.* **12,** 857–872.

Kraal, G., Weissman, I. L., and Butcher, E. C. (1983). *J. Immunol.* **130,** 1097–1102.

Kristensen, T., and Tack, B. F. (1986). *Proc. Natl. Acad. Sci. U.S.A.* **83,** 3963–3967.

Kurosawa, S., Stearns, D., Jackson, K., and Esmon, C. (1988). *J. Biol. Chem.* **263,** 5993–5996.

Kyte, J., and Doolittle, R. F. (1982). *J. Mol. Biol.* **157,** 105–132.

Larsen, E., Celi, A., Gilbert, G. E., Furie, B. C., Erban, J. K., Bonfanti, R., Wagner, D. D., and Furie, B. (1989). *Cell* **59,** 305–312.

Larsen, E., Palabrica, T., Sajer, S., Gilbert, G. E., Wagner, D. D., Furie, B. C., and Furie, B. (1990). *Cell* **63,** 467–474.

Lasky, L. A., Singer, M. S., Yednock, T. A., Dowbenko, D., Fennie, C., Rodriguez, H., Nguyen, T., Stachel, S., and Rosen, S. D. (1989). *Cell* **56,** 1045–1055.
Leonard, W. J., Depper, J. M., Kanehisa, M., Kronke, M., Peffer, N. J., Svetlik, P. B., Sullivan, M., and Greene, W. C. (1985). *Science* **230,** 633–639.
Lewinsohn, D. M., Bargatze, R. F., and Butcher, E. C. (1987). *J. Immunol.* **138,** 4313–4321.
Lipman, D. J., and Pearson, W. R. (1985). *Science* **227,** 1435–1441.
Lowe, J. B., Stoolman, L. M., Nair, R. P., Larsen, R. D., Berhend, T. L., and Marks, R. M. (1990). *Cell* **63,** 475–484.
Lozier, J., Takahashi, N., and Putnam, F. W. (1984). *Proc. Natl. Acad. Sci. U.S.A.* **81,** 3640–3644.
McEver, R. P., and Martin, M. N. (1984). *J. Biol. Chem.* **259,** 9799–9804.
Marchesi, V., and Gowans, J. (1964). *Philos. Trans. R. Soc. (London)* **B 159,** 283.
Paulson, J. (1985). *In* "The Receptors" (P. Conn, ed), pp. 131–219. Academic Press, New York.
Pearse, B. M. (1988). *Embo. J.* **7,** 3331–3336.
Phillips, M. L., Nudelman, E., Gaeta, F. C., Perez, M., Singhal, A. K., Hakomori, S., and Paulson, J. C. (1990). *Science* **250,** 1130–1132.
Picker, L. J., de los Toyos, J., Telen, M. J., Haynes, B. F., and Butcher, E. C. (1989). *J. Immunol.* **142,** 2046–2051.
Rasmussen, R. A., Chin, Y. H., Woodruff, J. J., and Easton, T. G. (1985). *J. Immunol.* **135,** 19–24.
Reichert, R. A., Gallatin, W. M., Butcher, E. C., and Weissman, I. L. (1984). *Cell* **38,** 89–99.
Reichert, R. A., Gallatin, W. M., Weissman, I. L., and Butcher, E. C. (1983). *J. Exp. Med.* **157,** 813–827.
Reichert, R. A., Jerabek, L., Gallatin, W. M., Butcher, E. C., and Weissman, I. L. (1986). *J. Immunol.* **136,** 3535–3542.
Reid, K. B., and Day, A. J. (1989). *Immunol. Today* **10,** 177–180.
Rice, M. C., and O'Brien, S. J. (1980). *Nature* **283,** 157–161.
Roths, J. B., Murphy, E. D., and Eicher, E. M. (1984). *J. Exp. Med.* **159,** 1–20.
Seldin, M. F., Morse, H. C., LeBoeuf, R. C., and Steinberg, A. D. (1988a). *Genomics* **2,** 48–56.
Seldin, M. F., Morse, H. C., Reeves, J. P., Scribner, C. L., LeBoeuf, R. C., and Steinberg, A. D. (1988b). *J. Exp. Med.* **167,** 688–693.
Sher, B. T., Bargatze, R., Holzmann, B., Gallatin, W. M., Matthews, D., Wu, N., Picker, L., Butcher, E. C., and Weissman, I. L. (1988). *Adv. Cancer. Res.* **51,** 361–390.
Siegelman, M., Bond, M. W., Gallatin, W. M., St, J. T., Smith, H. T., Fried, V. A., and Weissman, I. L. (1986). *Science* **231,** 823–829.
Siegelman, M. H., Cheng, I. C., Weissman, I. L., and Wakeland, E. K. (1990). *Cell* **61,** 611–622.
Siegelman, M. H., van de Rijn, M., and Weissman, I. L. (1989). *Science* **243,** 1165–1172.
Siegelman, M. H., and Weissman, I. L. (1989). *Proc. Natl. Acad. Sci. U.S.A.* **86,** 5562–5566.
Singer, P. A., McEvilly, R. J., Balderas, R. S., Dixon, F. J., and Theofilopoulos, A. N. (1988). *Proc. Natl. Acad. Sci. U.S.A.* **85,** 7729–7733.
Spiess, M., and Lodish, H. F. (1985). *Proc. Natl. Acad. Sci. U.S.A.* **82,** 6465–6469.
Spiess, M., Schwartz, A. L., and Lodish, H. F. (1985). *J. Biol. Chem.* **260,** 1979–1982.
St. John, T., Gallatin, W. M., Siegelman, M., Smith, H. T., Fried, V. A., and Weissman, I. L. (1986). *Science* **231,** 845–850.
St. John, T., Meyer, J., Idzerda, R., and Gallatin, W. M. (1990). *Cell* **60,** 45–52.
Stamenkovic, I., Amiot, M., Pesando, J. M., and Seed, B. (1989). *Cell* **56,** 1057–1062.
Stamper, H. J., and Woodruff, J. J. (1976). *J. Exp. Med.* **144,** 828–833.
Stevens, S. K., Weissman, I. L., and Butcher, E. C. (1982). *J. Immunol.* **128,** 844–851.
Stoolman, L. M. (1989). *Cell* **56,** 907–910.
Stoolman, L. M., and Rosen, S. D. (1983). *J. Cell. Biol.* **96,** 722–729.
Stoolman, L. M., Tenforde, T. S., and Rosen, S. D. (1984). *J. Cell. Biol.* **99,** 1.
Stoolman, L. M., Yednock, T. A., and Rosen, S. D. (1987). *Blood* **70,** 1842–1850.

Streeter, P. R., Berg, E. L., Rouse, B. T., Bargatze, R. F., and Butcher, E. C. (1988). *Nature (London)* **331,** 41–46.

Tada, N., Kimura, S., Liu, L. Y., and Hammerling, U. (1983). *Hybridoma* **2,** 29–38.

Takada, S., Koide, J., and Engleman, E. G. (1989). *J. Immunol.* **142,** 3038–3044.

Tedder, T. F., Isaacs, C. M., Ernst, T. J., Demetri, G. D., Adler, D. A., and Disteche, C. M. (1989). *J. Exp. Med.* **170,** 123–133.

Tiemeyer, M., Swiedler, S. J., Ishihara, M., Moreland, M., Schweingruber, H., Hirtzer, P., and Brandley, B. K. (1991). *Proc. Natl. Acad. Sci. U.S.A.* **88,** 1138–1142.

Trowbridge, I. S., Lesley, J., Schulte, R., Hyman, R., and Trotter, J. (1982). *Immunogenetics* **15,** 299–312.

van de Rijn, M., Weissman, I. L., and Siegelman, M. (1990). *J. Immunol.* **145,** 1477–1482.

Walz, G., Aruffo, A., Kolanus, W., Bevilacqua, M., and Seed, B. (1990). *Science* **250,** 1132–1135.

Watson, J., Kingsmore, S., Johnston, G., Siegelman, M., Le Beau, M., Lemons, R., Bora, N. S., Howard, T., Weissman, I., McEver, R., and Seldin, M. (1990). *J. Exp. Med.* **172,** 263.

Weissman, I. L. (1967). *J. Exp. Med.* **126,** 291–304.

Weissman, I. L., Baird, S., Gardner, R., Papaioannou, V., and Raschke, W. (1977). *Cold Spring Harbor Symp. Quant. Biol.* **41,** 9–21.

Weissman, I. L., Gutman, G. A., and Friedberg, S. H. (1974). *Ser. Haematol.* **7,** 482–504.

Wharton, K. A., Johansen, K. M., Xu, T., and Artavanis, T. S. (1985). *Cell*

Wiley, D. C., and Skehel, J. J. (1987). *Annu. Rev. Biochem.*

Woodruff, J. J., Clarke, L. M., and Chin, Y. H. (1987). *Annu. Rev. Immunol.* **5,** 201–222.

Yednock, T. A., Butcher, E. C., Stoolman, L. M., and Rosen, S. D. (1987). *J. Cell. Biol.* **104,** 725–731.

Yednock, T. A., and Rosen, S. D. (1989). *Adv. Immunol.* **44,** 313–378.

Yednock, T. A., Stoolman, L. M., and Rosen, S. D. (1987b). *J. Cell. Biol.* **104,** 713–723.

CHAPTER 5

The Peyer's Patch Homing Receptor: A Novel Member of the Integrin Family

Mickey C-T. Hu, Bernhard Holzmann, Heinz Neuhaus, and Irving L. Weissman

Howard Hughes Medical Institute
Departments of Pathology and Developmental Biology
Stanford University School of Medicine
Stanford, California 94305

I. Introduction

Most mature lymphocytes, but not other blood borne cells, continuously recirculate from blood through secondary lymphoid organs and back into the bloodstream (Gowans and Knight, 1964). The traffic of lymphocytes throughout the body, among various lymphoid organs, is not random but is a well-orchestrated process that enables the immunocompetent lymphocytes to be efficiently deployed. It confers the dynamic control of distribution of the antigen reactive repertoire that is available to encounter appropriately processed antigen at any site in the body, regardless of which portal mediates its entry. When lymphocytes enter various lymphoid organs, they are exposed to an array of antigen-presenting cells and

Cellular and Molecular Mechanisms of Inflammation, Volume 2

are, therefore, stimulated to become activated and multiply if their specific antigen is currently present in the body. This migratory behavior of lymphocytes is also thought to be critical in disseminating locally activated effector cells and memory populations to distant lymphoid organs and sites of inflammation. To enter lymphoid organs, lymphocytes extravasate from the blood by adhering to and migrating through specialized high endothelial venules (HEVs) via adhesion molecules termed homing receptors (Stamper and Woodruff, 1976); whereas to enter inflammatory sites, lymphocytes adhere to and migrate through transiently activated endothelium, which is probably stimulated by local release of inflammatory mediators in the inflamed tissue. Thus far, as shown in Fig. 1, at least three functionally and antigenically distinct lymphocyte-HEV recognition systems governing the homing of lymphocytes to peripheral lymph nodes, mucosal lymphoid organs (Peyer's patches or appendix), and inflamed synovium have been identified (for reviews, see Gallatin *et al.*, 1986; Jalkanen *et al.*, 1986; Stoolman, 1989). The highly organ specific interactions of lymphocytes with HEVs are believed to be controlled by homing receptors on lymphocytes and vascular addressins on HEVs (Streeter *et al.*, 1988a,b). The murine lymph node-specific homing receptor is defined by antibody MEL-14, which recognizes a branched-chain ubiquitinated glycoprotein on the surface of lymphocytes with an apparent

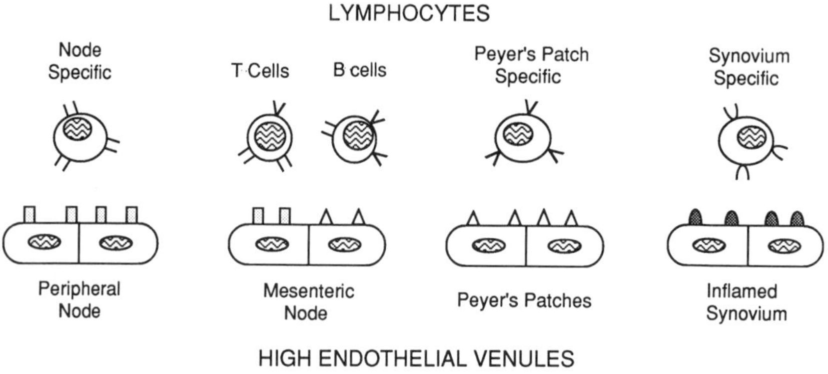

FIGURE 1

Proposed model of complementary receptors on lymphocytes and HEV. Three distinct lymphocyte homing receptors and their specific complementary ligands are depicted, one expressed on peripheral lymph node HEV, one on Peyer's patch HEV, and one on inflamed synovium. Both peripheral node- and Peyer's patch-specific ligands are expressed on mesenteric lymph node HEV, which bind both peripheral node- and Peyer's patch-specific lymphocytes.

molecular weight of ~90 kDa (reviewed by Gallatin *et al.*, 1986), and its cDNA has been cloned and well characterized (Siegelman *et al.*, 1989; Lasky *et al.*, 1989). Furthermore, a cDNA clone encoding the human homologue of this homing receptor has been isolated and characterized (Siegelman and Weissman, 1989; Tedder *et al.*, 1989).

The murine lymphocyte Peyer's patch specific adhesion molecules (LPAM) involved in the tissue specific adhesion of lymphocytes to Peyer's patch HEV have been identified to be members of the integrin family of adhesion receptors (Holzmann *et al.*, 1989; Holzmann and Weissman, 1989a,b). LPAM-1 consists of an integrin α subunit (α_{4m}) with a molecular weight of ~150 kDa homologous to the human α_4 (VLA-4α) and a novel integrin β subunit (designated as β_p) with a molecular weight of ~130 kDa, whereas LPAM-2 consists of the same α_{4m} subunit and the integrin β_1 subunit (Holzmann and Weissman, 1989a). Although LPAM-2 may also mediate adhesion to Peyer's patch HEVs, it is not likely to be organ-specific because the human $\alpha_4\beta_1$ molecule has multiple other functions (Hemler *et al.*, 1990). Perhaps LPAM-2 requires other accessory molecules to facilitate its attachment to Peyer's patch HEVs because it is also present on some nonbinding lymphoma cells that do not home to Peyer's patches. The association of LPAM α and β heterodimers requires the presence of Ca^{2+} ions.

Generally speaking, the integrin family of adhesion receptors are engaged in various aspects of cellular adhesion and interactions with extracellular matrix (ECM) components (reviewed by Hynes 1987; Ruoslahti and Pierschbacher, 1987). The integrin family consists of at least 11 different α subunits and 7 different β subunits that are associated to form at least 14 different $\alpha\beta$ heterodimers, currently divided into three subfamilies according to distinct β subunits (for reviews, see Kishimoto *et al.*, 1989; Ruoslahti and Giancotti, 1989; Hemler, 1990; Hemler *et al.*, 1990; Larson and Springer, 1990; Springer, 1990). The integrin β_1 subfamily (the VLA subfamily containing at least six distinct members) and β_3 subfamily [the cytoadhesin subfamily containing the vitronectin receptor ($\alpha_v\beta_3$) and platelet glycoprotein IIb/IIIa ($\alpha_{IIb}\beta_3$)] have been shown to be involved directly in cell adhesion to ECM components including collagen, fibronectin, and laminin. Integrin members of these two subfamilies appear to play an important role in hemostasis, growth and repair, and embryogenesis. The β_2 subfamily (the Leu-CAM subfamily containing LFA-1, Mac-1, and p150,95) have been found to mediate various aspects of leukocyte adhesion, giving them a crucial role in inflammatory and immune responses (reviewed by Kishimoto *et al.*, 1989; Springer, 1990). Initially, only three different β subunits had been identified, β_1, β_2, and β_3. Therefore, the three subfamilies are thought to contain multiple heterodimers and each heterodimer consists of a common β subunit associated with several distinct α subunits, which provide ligand specificity, whereas each α subunit associates with only one β subunit. However, several α subunits have been found to associate with multiple β subunits since four additional (or alternative) β subunits have been identified, namely β_4 (Kajiji *et al.*, 1989; Hemler *et al.*, 1989), β_5 (or β_x) (Cheresh *et al.*, 1989; Ramaswamy and Hemler, 1990), β_s (Freed *et al.*, 1989), β_p (Holzmann and Weissman, 1989a), and β_6 (Sheppard *et al.*, 1990). For example, α_6 can associate with both β_1 and β_4 (Hemler *et al.*, 1989; Kajiji *et al.*, 1989), α_v can associate with β_3, β_5, β_s (Cheresh *et al.*, 1989), and α_4 can associate with both β_1 and β_p (Holzmann and Weissman, 1989a).

II. Structure of LPAM-1: A Novel Integrin Molecule $\alpha_4\beta_p$

A. The α_4 Subunit

A murine cDNA clone encoding the integrin α_4 subunit (designated as α_{4m}) has been isolated and characterized (Neuhaus *et al.*, 1991). The sequence of this cDNA encodes a peptide of 1039 amino acids and shows a 84% homology with the human α_4 subunit (VLA-4α). The primary structure of the α_{4m} subunit is very similar to that of human α_4 subunit (reviewed by Hemler, 1990). Like other integrin α subunits, the α_{4m} contains a short carboxylterminal cytoplasmic domain, a single transmembrane domain, and a large extracellular domain. The extracellular domain of α_{4m}contains three putative divalent cation binding regions of the general structure DXDXDGXXD. Although the integrin α subunits exhibit more sequence heterogeneity (17 to 24% homology) than the β subunits (See Section B), these putative divalent cation binding regions are among the most conserved sequences between the α_{4m} and other known α subunits, suggesting that they may be involved in the association of α and β subunits. Unlike the Leu-CAM and VLA-2 α subunits containing an additional amino acid sequence inserted between the aminoterminus and the last divalent cation binding region (the "I" domain), α_{4m} does not contain an "I" domain. The positions of the characteristic cysteine residues are conserved between the α_{4m} and human α_4. Unlike other integrin α subunits, a putative protease cleavage site is located about the middle of the α_{4m} peptide sequence. This cleavage will yield fragments of ~80 kDa and ~70 kDa, which have been shown by our previous immunoprecipitation data (Holzmann *et al.*, 1989).

B. The β_p Subunit

A murine full-length cDNA clone encoding the novel integrin β_p subunit has been isolated and characterized (Hu *et al.*, in preparation). The sequence of this cDNA encodes an 806 amino acid potentially highly glycosylated transmembrane protein. Its sequence is unique but shows significant homology with those of the other integrin β subunits, suggesting that it is a new member of the integrin family of adhesion receptors. The β subunits of all known integrins are markedly similar. The predicted amino acid sequence of this novel β_p subunit is most related to human integrin β_2 (49% overall identity), and to a lesser extent, related to β_1 (45% identity), β_5 (40% identity), β_3 (39% identity), β_6 (39% identity), and β_4 (34% idenity).

Although the gross structure of the β_p subunit is similar to that of the other integrin β subunits, it has two unique features. One major difference is that only 54 cysteine residues present in the extracellular domain of the β_p subunit are conserved with the other integrin β subunits except the β_4 subunit, which lacks 6 of the 54 conserved cysteines. However, all 56 cysteine residues in the integrin β_1, β_2, β_3, β_5, β_6 subunits from human and the integrin β_1 subunits from mouse (Tominaga, 1988; Holers *et al.*, 1989), chicken (Tamkun *et al.*, 1986), *Xenopus* (DeSimone and Hynes, 1988), and *Drosophila* (MacKrell *et al.*, 1988) are present in the extracellular domain and fully conserved. On the other hand, there is a cysteine residue present in the predicted transmembrane domain of the β_p subunit that is absent from all of the other integrin β subunits. The other major difference is that the β_p subunit contains two extra hydrophobic regions near the transmembrane domain (Fig. 2B), residues 634 to 663 and 675 to 691 of the predicted mature protein (Hu *et al.*, in preparation). These are absent from all of the other known integrin β subunits. It is not known whether or not these two hydrophobic regions can form two membrane spanning domains. If they do, the structure of this novel β_p subunit will be very distinct from other known integrin β subunits. In general, the transmembrane domain is not significantly conserved and the cytoplasmic domain is weakly conserved among those β subunits. The cytoplasmic domain of the β_p subunit is slightly longer than those of the other β subunits except the β_4 subunit, which contains a very large (ca. 1000 amino acids) cytoplasmic domain.

There are three tyrosine residues at positions 733, 738, and 758 in the cytoplasmic domain of β_p. Tyrosine 733 located six amino acids downstream from a basic residue (arginine) and two amino acids downstream from an acidic residue (glutamic acid), and tyrosine 758 located seven amino acids downstream from a basic residue (lysine) and five amino

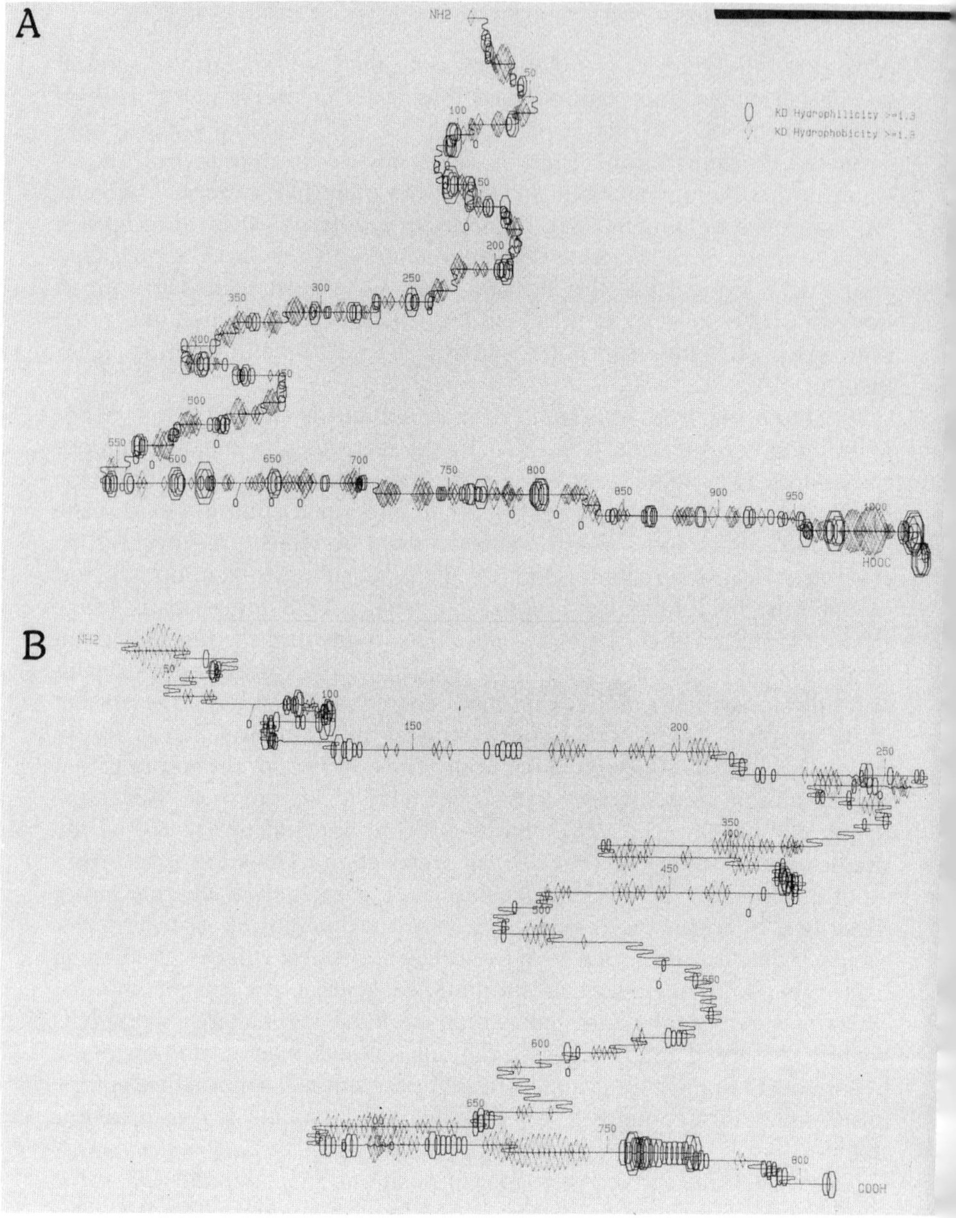
A
NH2
KD Hydrophilicity >=1.3
KD Hydrophobicity >=1.3
HOOC
B
NH2
COOH

acids downstream from an acidic residue (aspartic acid); these fit features characteristic for tyrosine kinase phosphorylation sites (Hunter and Cooper, 1985). In particular, the sequences around tyrosine 758 of the β_p subunit are conserved with the β_1, β_3, and β_5 subunits, with a consensus sequence NPLYK, and show a degree of homology with tyrosine kinase phosphorylation sites in the EGF receptor, insulin receptor, and neu oncogene protein, as described previously (Tamkun *et al.*, 1986). In the β_4 subunit, however, a tyrosine residue (residue 1668) with the homologous sequence NVPYK near the C-terminal can be a potential site for tyrosine phosphorylation (Hogervorst *et al.*, 1990; Suzuki and Naitoh, 1990). Interestingly, the sequences near the tyrosine 758 of the β_p subunit match the consensus sequence NPXY/F required for receptor-mediated endocytosis (Chen *et al.*, 1990), which are also conserved in these integrin β subunits except the β_4 subunit.

A striking feature of the β_p subunit is the arrangement of its cysteine residues in the extracellular domain. Between amino acids 459 and 632, the β_p subunit contains four tandem repeats of cysteine rich motifs with small gaps, each with eight cysteines (seven in the first repeat) in a conserved configuration (Fig. 3A). Comparison of these cysteine rich motifs of β_p to sequences in the NBRF database revealed many proteins that contain similar sequence motifs and the conserved arrangement of cysteines. The first protein described with this sequence motif is the epidermal growth factor (EGF) precursor, which contains ten homologous copies (Gray *et al.*, 1983; Scott *et al.*, 1983). Fig. 3B shows the sequences of proteins with the EGF-like domains that are homologous to these cysteine rich motifs of β_p. It is generally believed that extracellular cysteines are disulfide bonded. Because there are no disulfide links between the α_{4m} and β_p subunits of LPAM-1, these conserved cysteines within the EGF-like domain should be involved in intrachain disulfide bonds, which should give the tandem EGF-like domains a very unique and rigid tertiary structure. The con-

FIGURE 2

The best predicted secondary structures of α_{4m} (A) and β_p (B). The computer program "Plotstructure" (Wolf *et al.*, 1987) generates a two-dimensional plot representing predicted secondary structures (helices, beta sheets, turns, and coils) with different wave forms. Helices are shown with a sine wave, beta sheets with a sharp saw-tooth wave, turns with 180 degree turns, and coils with a dull saw-tooth wave. Hydrophilicity (◯, ≥1.3) and hydrophobicity (◊, ≥1.3) are superimposed over the wave with special symbols as indicated. The size of the symbols is proportional to the value of the attribute. Possible glycosylation sites are marked with an open circle below the wave.

sensus sequence for EGF-like domains includes at least six conserved cysteine residues that can form three disulfide bridges (Cooke *et al.*, 1987). The homologies per se and available functional data suggest that these domains share some common functional features.

Several lines of evidence suggest that proteins containing one or more EGF-like domains are directly involved in protein–protein or receptor–ligand interactions. Firstly, EGF is a 53-residue, three-disulfide bridged, single-chain polypeptide that binds to a specific cell surface receptor having cytoplasmic tyrosine-kinase activity that mediates its mitogenic and pleiotropic proliferative activities (reviewed by Carpenter and Cohen,

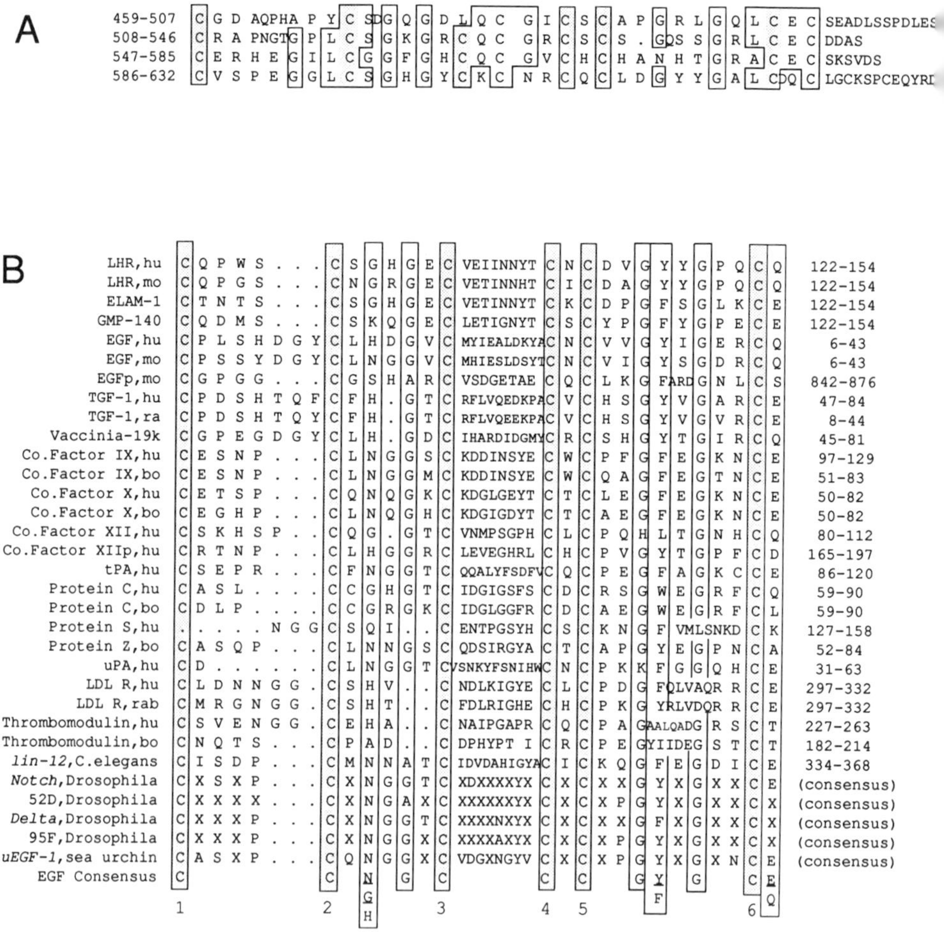

1979). Certain shorter synthetic peptides compete with authentic EGF for receptor binding and mimic some of the functions of EGF, indicating that the minimal receptor binding sequence lies within residues 20 to 31 (Komoriya *et al.*, 1984). However, shorter synthetic peptides containing this minimal receptor binding region have much less affinity for the receptor than authentic EGF (Heath and Merrifield, 1986), suggesting that the tertiary structure of EGF contributes to its receptor binding affinity. Secondly, urokinase-type plasminogen activator (uPA) binds to its receptor with high affinity through its N-terminal region (residues 1 to 135), which contains an EGF-like domain (Stoppelli *et al.*, 1985). Synthetic peptide studies show that the receptor binding specificity locates within residues 18 to 32 of uPA (i.e., within the EGF-like domain) (Appella *et al.*, 1987). Thirdly, the B1 chain of laminin appears to be involved in binding to collagen and to cell surface receptors. The sequence of this molecule encodes several EGF-like, cysteine rich repeats. Synthetic peptide studies have shown that residues 925 to 933 of this polypeptide in one of these EGF-like domains is mainly responsible for the receptor-binding, cell attachment and migration activities of laminin (Graf *et al.*, 1987). Fourthly, the LDL receptor contains three copies of EGF-like repeats in the extracellular domain. Structural analysis of the LDL-receptor gene reveals that deletion of exons 7 and 8 (i.e., the first two copies of the EGF-like repeat)

FIGURE 3

Alignment of the tandemly repeated EGF-like domains in β_P with similar domains in other proteins. (A) Homologous repeats of an EGF-like motif in the β_P subunit were aligned with the BESTFIT program of the GCG software package of the University of Wisconsin (Devereux *et al.*, 1984). The numbers to the left of the sequence are the residue numbers for β_P. Homologous residues are boxed. (B) Homologous sequences from vertebrates and invertebrates, in the protein sequence databank, containing the characteristic EGF-like motif are compared. The numbers to the right of the sequence indicate the residue numbers for the proteins where these homologous sequences are located. Dots denote gaps introduced to gain optimal alignment. The boxed residues indicate homologous matches to the consensus sequence of the EGF-like domain and the shaded boxes show the positions of conserved cysteine residues in this domain. hu, human; mo, mouse; ra, rat; bo, bovine; rab, rabbit; p, precursor; LHR, lymph node homing receptor; ELAM, endothelial adhesion molecule; GMP, granule membrane protein; EGF, epidermal growth factor; TGF, transforming growth factor; Vaccinia, Vaccinia virus; Co. Factor, Coagulation Factor; tPA, tissue plasminogen activator; uPA, urokinase-type plasminogen activator; LDL R, low density lipoprotein receptor; uEGF-1, and EGF homolog in sea urchins.

strongly interferes with the ligand binding capacity and specificity of this receptor (Yamamoto *et al.*, 1986). In addition to the binding of LDL, these EGF-like domains appear to allow the receptor to engage in repeated recycling without degradation (Davis *et al.*, 1987). Fifthly, thrombomodulin is an endothelial cell surface glycoprotein that contains six tandemly repeated EGF-like domains. A fragment of thrombomodulin containing the fifth and sixth EGF-like repeats has been proposed to act as the primary thrombin binding site (Kurosawa *et al.*, 1988). Sixthly, as illustrated in Fig. 3B, many other proteins containing one or more EGF-like domains are cell adhesion molecules, growth factors, receptors or receptor-like proteins, and proteins of the coagulation and fibrinolytic pathway, suggesting that the EGF-like domains are generally involved in protein–protein or receptor–ligand interactions. Finally and perhaps most significantly, the lymph node homing receptor core protein contains an EGF-like domain close to its lectin-binding domain in the extracellular region that is conserved between mouse and human (Siegelman *et al.*, 1989; Lasky *et al.*, 1989; Siegelman and Weissman, 1989; Tedder *et al.*, 1989). Sequence analysis of the allelic determinant of this homing receptor (Ly-22) shows a single amino acid interchange within this EGF-like domain. In the HEV frozen section assay (the *in vitro* binding assay), anti-Ly-22 antibody strongly inhibits attachment of lymphocytes to HEVs but does not block MEL-14 antibody binding to the adjacent lectin domain, suggesting that this EGF-like domain is directly involved in the adhesion of lymphocytes to lymph node HEVs (Siegelman *et al.*, 1990).

C. Structure of LPAM-1

The structure of LPAM-1 is predicted by our knowledge of integrin structure, which is primarily based on extensive biochemical studies of the platelet membrane glycoprotein $gpII_b/III_a$ ($\alpha II_b\beta_3$) complex (Phillips *et al.*, 1988), and the best predicted secondary structures of α_{4m} (Fig. 2A) and β_p (Fig. 2B). A schematic representation of a possible structure of LPAM-1 is illustrated in Fig. 4. An association of the amino-portion globular domains of the α and β subunits to form the extracellular ligand binding regions of the receptor has been suggested by electron microscopic images of purified integrins (Nermut *et al.*, 1988) as well as chemical cross-linking experiments (Smith and Cheresh, 1988; D'Souza *et al.*, 1988). Furthermore, biochemical analysis of the integrin β_3 subunit (Beer and Coller, 1989) suggests that the aminoterminal portion of the β subunit is folded into a loop that is stabilized by disulfide bonds formed between cysteines near the aminoterminus portion and those within the first cysteine rich repeat (EGF-like domain).

As the association of the α_{4m} and β_p subunits requires the presence of Ca^{2+} (Holzmann *et al.*, 1989), it is reasonable to propose that one function of Ca^{2+} ions is to maintain the structural integrity of LPAM-1, the association of α_{4m} and β_p, via heterodimer. The α_{4m} subunit contains three tandem repeats of about 60 amino acids in the extracellular domain having putative divalent cation binding sites (Neuhaus *et al.*, submitted). As shown in Fig. 5, sequence analysis for the β_p cDNA clone has also revealed one EF loop (or EF-hand loop) consensus sequence (Vyas *et al.*, 1987; reviewed by Strynadka and James, 1989), residues 158 to 169, that is a potential Ca^{2+} binding site on β_p. Alteration of the EF loop (Ca^{2+} binding site) of the β_3 subunit by site-directed mutagenesis appears to diminish ligand binding to the mutant $\alpha II_b\beta_3$, suggesting that this region may be directly involved in ligand binding (Loftus *et al.*, 1990). If this is a common mechanism of ligand binding for integrin receptors, this EF loop sequence motif may not be involved in the association of the α_{4m} and β_p subunits. Instead, as proposed in Fig. 4, the α_{4m} and β_p subunits may be bridged with Ca^{2+} ions between divalent cation binding sites on α_{4m} and the EGF-like domains on β_p because these domains have been implicated to carry a high-affinity Ca^{2+} binding site (Handford *et al.*, 1990).

Many studies (Argraves *et al.*, 1989; Buck *et al.*, 1986; Burridge *et al.*, 1988; Solowska *et al.*, 1989) have shown that integrin binding to the cytoskeleton requires the cytoplasmic domain of the β subunit. The association of integrins with cytoskeletal proteins has been demonstrated to be via an indirect linkage, involving fibulin, talin, vinculin, and perhaps other cytoskeletal proteins (Burridge *et al.*, 1988). Although the cytoplasmic domain of the β_1 subunit is highly conserved among human (Argraves *et al.*, 1987), mouse (Tominaga, 1988; Holers *et al.*, 1989), chicken (Tamkun *et al.*, 1986), *Xenopus* (DeSimone and Hynes, 1988), and *Drosophila* (MacKrell *et al.*, 1988), it is one of the least conserved regions among different integrin β subunits, with regard to sequence homology and the length of this domain in all subunits. This evident dissimilarity among the cytoplasmic domains of various integrin β subunits suggests that each β subunit may be involved in a specialized function, perhaps via unique cytoskeletal elements. Tyrosine phosphorylation within the cytoplasmic domain of integrin β subunits are thought to play an important regulatory role in integrin function (Hirst *et al.*, 1986). Amino acid sequence analysis for a variety of integrin molecules has revealed a potential site for tyrosine phosphorylation in the cytoplasmic domain of most of the α (Takada *et al.*, 1989; Neuhaus *et al.*, 1991) and β subunits, with the homologous sequences KRQYK and NPLYK, respectively. Interestingly, it has been reported that each α subunit of the Leu-CAM molecules (CD11/CD18 leukocyte integrin subfamily) is constitutively phosphorylated in the cells in which it is expressed whereas the β subunit (β_2, in this case) is not phosphorylated in resting cells but becomes strongly phosphorylated in cells stimulated with phorbol 12-myristate 13-acetate (PMA) (Buyon *et al.*, 1990). The constitutive phosphorylation of the α subunits and the conditional phosphorylation of the β subunits upon induction with stimulus may be governed by the distinct recognition sequences for the potential phosphorylation sites in each subunit, by different kinases, or both. However, the functional role of these potential phosphorylations in the integrin α and β subunits remains to be established.

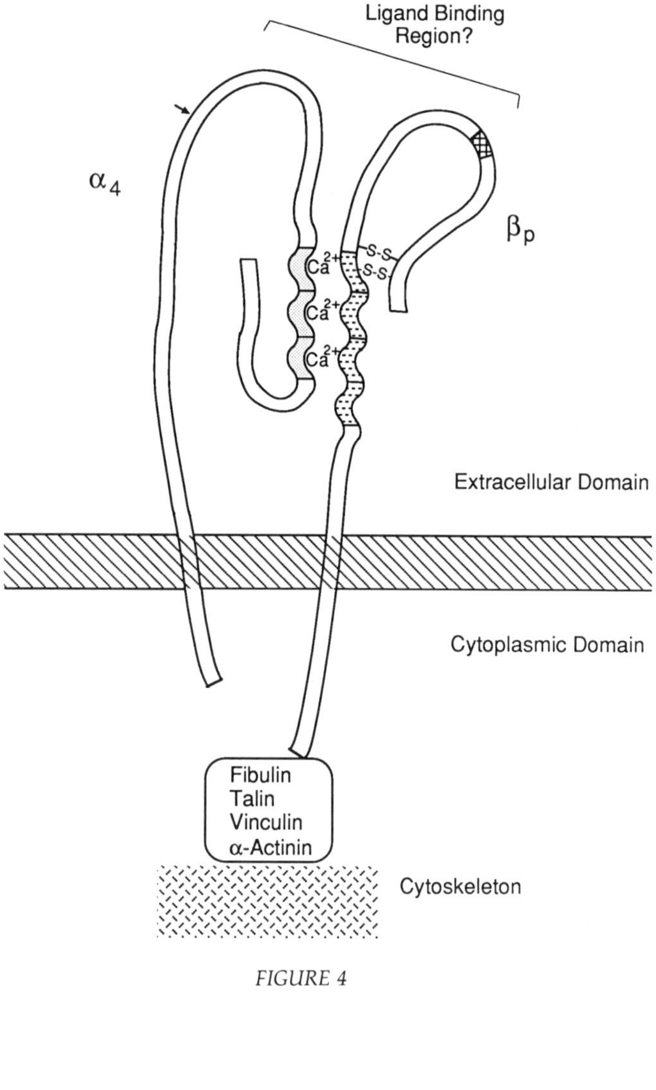

FIGURE 4

βp	D	L	S	Y	S	M	K	D	D	L	E	R
β1	D	L	S	Y	S	M	K	D	D	L	E	N
β2	D	L	S	Y	S	M	I	D	D	L	R	N
β3	D	L	S	Y	S	M	K	D	D	L	W	S
β4	D	F	S	N	S	M	S	D	D	L	D	N
β5	D	L	S	L	S	M	K	D	D	L	D	N
β6	D	L	S	A	S	M	D	D	D	L	N	T
Avian β1	D	L	S	Y	S	M	K	D	D	L	E	N
Frog β1	D	L	S	F	S	M	K	D	D	L	E	N
Dro.mys	D	L	S	K	S	M	E	D	D	K	A	K
EF loop	X		Y		Z		-Y		-X			-Z

FIGURE 5

Alignment of the region of the β_p subunit containing the EF loop consensus sequence (residues 158 to 169) with other integrin β subunits. The aligned amino acid sequences (one-letter code) are from human β_1, β_2, β_3, β_4, β_5, β_6, avian β_1, frog β_1, and *Drosophila melanogaster l*(1) *mys* (lethal myospheroid gene product). Oxygenated residues that align with those in the EF loop consensus sequence are boxed, and the most conserved oxygenated residues are shaded. The residues that may form the putative calcium coordination octahedron are labeled by X, Y, Z, -Y, -X, -Z.

FIGURE 4

Schematic representation of a possible structure of LPAM-1. LPAM-1 is composed of two noncovalently associated integrin α_4 and β_p subunits. Both subunits are integral membrane glycoproteins. The cell membrane is shown as a hatched region. The α_4 subunit contains three divalent cation binding domains that are denoted with shaded regions. A putative protease cleavage site is highlighted with an arrow. The β_p subunit contains four tandemly repeated, cysteine rich EGF-like domains (indicated with dashed regions) that may carry high-affinity Ca^{2+} binding sites (Handford *et al.*, 1990). The large loop in the aminoterminus portion of the extracellular domain of the β_p subunit may be stabilized by intrachain disulfide bonding (shown as -S-S-), which is supported by the evidence of the integrin β_3 subunit (Beer and Coller, 1989). The extracellular domains of α_4 and β_p should contain the ligand binding region. One EF loop (or EF-hand loop) domain, denoted as a small region with crossed lines, on the β_p subunit may be involved in the ligand binding region. The cytoplasmic domains of the α_4 subunit is relatively smaller than that of the β_p subunit that may be associated with cytoskeletal elements, including fibulin, talin, vinculin, and α-actinin, which link LPAM-1 to the cytoskeleton.

III. Tissue Distribution of LPAM-1

The distribution of the expression of RNA species encoding the β_p subunit is predominantly in lymphoid tissues, a finding that correlates well with the distribution of the α_{4m} subunit (Neuhaus *et al.*, 1991). While the integrin β_1 subunit is widely distributed on hematopoietic cells (Wayner *et al.*, 1989), it is also expressed at relatively high level in heart, kidney, brain, and lung (Holers *et al.*, 1989). In contrast, by Northern analysis, we show no detectable β_p transcripts in heart, muscle, and testis, and very low levels in kidney, brain, liver, and lung (Hu *et al.*, in preparation). The tissue distribution of other β subunits is still unknown. However, it has been documented that the β_2 integrin subunit is expressed exclusively on leukocytes (Kishimoto *et al.*, 1989) and the β_3 integrin subunit is expressed primarily in platelets (Phillips *et al.*, 1988). This implies that different cell types in different tissues (or organs) utilize different integrin molecules for adhesion function.

IV. LPAM-2 ($\alpha_{4m}\beta_1$): Another Receptor Involved in Lymphocyte Homing to Peyer's Patches?

We (Holzmann and Weissman, 1989a) have shown that LPAM-1 ($\alpha_{4m}\beta_p$) is invariantly but LPAM-2 ($\alpha_{4m}\beta_1$) is in one case (TK50 lymphoma cells) involved in lymphocyte homing to Peyer's patches. LPAM-2 is predominantly expressed on lymphoma cells that do not bind to Peyer's patch HEVs, suggesting that expression of LPAM-2 alone is not sufficient to mediate this adhesive event. Immunoprecipitation experiments using the anti-α_{4m} monoclonal antibody R1-2 show that no detectable level of β_p, and therefore LPAM-1 is expressed on TK50 lymphoma cells. It is tempting to postulate that one or more adhesion molecules, including H-CAM (Pgp-1), LFA-1, etc., may operate concurrently with LPAM-2 to mediate adhesion of lymphocytes to Peyer's patch HEVs (see below). Although the LFA-1 molecule has been suggested to function as an accessory molecule in lymphocyte homing to lymph nodes and Peyer's patches (Hamann *et al.*, 1988; Pals *et al.*, 1988), it is unlikely to be the only functional accessory molecule for LPAM-2 to bind to Peyer's patch HEVs, because it is generally expressed on LPAM-2$^+$ nonbinding lymphomas. It is still possible that TK50 lymphoma cells may express low but functional levels of LPAM-1 not detectable by immunoprecipitation experiments performed with anti-α_{4m} monoclonal antibody R1-2. Alternatively, if LPAM-2 is a homing receptor for inflamed HEV in mucosal lymphoid organs, TK50 lymphoma cells might bind to the inflammatory component(s) on Peyer's patch HEV.

V. Accessory Molecules for Lymphocyte Homing to Peyer's Patches

In humans, a lymphocyte surface glycoprotein(s) of ~90 kDa ($gp90^{Hermes}$) defined by the Hermes series of monoclonal antibodies is reported to be involved in lymphocyte organ specific adhesion to lymph node, mucosal, or synovial HEVs (Jalkanen *et al.*, 1986, 1987). The lymphocyte Hermes antigen $gp90^{Hermes}$ has been shown to be identical to CD44 and human Pgp-1 antigens (Goldstein *et al.*, 1989; Idzerda *et al.*, 1989; Picker *et al.*, 1989). In the mouse, however, expression of the homologue of this antigen (Pgp-1 or H-CAM or Ly-24) alone appears not to be sufficient for lymphocyte organ specific adhesion to Peyer's patch HEVs (Table I). Nei-

TABLE I

Adhesion Molecules that May Be Involved in Lymphocyte-Binding to Peyer's Patch HEV

Cells	Binding to PP-HEV[a]	Inhibition by R1-2	LPAM-1 (α_{4m}/β_p)[b]	LPAM-2 (α_{4m}/β_1)	H-CAM (Pgp-1)[c]
MLN cells	++	+++	+	+	+
TK1 (T)	+++	+++	+	–	+
TK23 (T)	+++	++	+	+	+
TK40 (T)	+++	+++	+	+	+
TK50 (T)	++	+++	–	+	+
KKT2 (T)	–	NA	–	+	+
RAW112 (B)	–	NA	–	+	+
T69 (B)	–	NA	–	+	+
L1-2 (B)	–	NA	–	+	–
TK5 (T)	–	NA	–	–	+
BW5147 (T)	–	NA	–	–	+

[a]The binding of lymphocytes to Peyer's patch HEV and the capacity of antibody R1-2 to inhibit lymphocyte adhesion to Peyer's patch HEV was determined by the *in vitro* HEV binding assay as described by Stamper and Woodruff (1976) and Butcher *et al.* (1979). Levels of inhibition are indicated by ++ (50 to 75%), +++ (75 to 100%), and – (no inhibition). NA = not applicable.

[b]Lymphocytes were surface iodinated and lysates were immunoprecipitated with antibody R1-2 covalently linked to Affigel 15 as described by Holzmann *et al.* (1989). Bound proteins were eluted at pH 2.5 and eluates were neutralized by dilution in 50 mM Tris pH 8.8, 150 mM NaCl, 10 mM EDTA, and 1% Triton X-100. Dissociated subunits were precipitated with different heteroantisera recognizing integrin β_1 or β_p or with control antibodies. Immunoprecipitates were analyzed by SDS-PAGE.

[c]Lymphocytes were stained with anti-H-CAM (Pgp-1) monoclonal antibody IM781 and analyzed by the fluorescence activated cytometric sorter (FACS).

ther lymphoid cell lines (TK5 and BW5147) expressing H-CAM alone bind to Peyer's patch HEV; nor do lymphoid cell lines (KKT2, RAW112 and T69) expressing H-CAM and LPAM-2. This suggests that H-CAM may function as a nonorgan specific accessory molecule for lymphocyte adhesion because it is a widespread primary cell surface adhesion molecule (Carter and Wayner, 1988; Picker *et al.*, 1989; Kansas *et al.*, 1989). However, H-CAM appears not to be associated with LPAM-1 since neither monoclonal antibody R1-2 nor anti-LPAM-1 polyclonal antiserum could immunoprecipitate H-CAM with α_{4m}, even if the cells had been treated with cross-linking reagents sufficient to couple α_{4m} and β_p (Holzmann *et al.*, 1989; Holzmann and Weissman, 1989a). Further experiments are investigating the topographical relationship between H-CAM and LPAM-1.

Antibodies to human or mouse LFA-1 partially inhibit lymphocyte-HEV interactions (Hamann *et al.*, 1988; Pals *et al.*, 1988), suggesting that LFA-1 may be involved in lymphocyte recirculation and homing. However, this inhibitory effect of anti-LFA-1 antibodies is virtually nonorgan specific, suggesting that the role of LFA-1 molecule in lymphocyte migration and homing is accessory.

VI. Possible Ligands for LPAM-1 or LPAM-2

The human VLA-4 ($\alpha_4\beta_1$) integrin has been shown to mediate adhesion of lymphocytes to IL-1 or TNF-α activated endothelial cells by binding to an inducible endothelial cell surface molecule termed VCAM-1 (Elices *et al.*, 1990). Also, $\alpha_4\beta_1$ has been shown to bind to the CS-1 domain of fibronectin that is distinct from the RGD (arg-gly-asp) adhesion sequence (Wayner *et al.*, 1989; Garcia-Pardo *et al.*, 1990; Davis *et al.*, 1990; Nojima *et al.*, 1990). The sites on VLA-4 involved in VCAM-1 binding are probably distinct from those involved in fibronectin binding. The sequence of VACM-1 indicates that it is a member of the immunoglobulin superfamily that appears to function in leukocyte–endothelial adhesion (Osborn *et al.*, 1989). It appears to be identical to an inducible 110-kDa endothelial cell adhesion molecule called INCAM-110 that mediates binding of some melanoma cells to activated endothelial cells (Rice and Bevilacqua, 1989). Interestingly, a new glycoprotein of 107 kDa that mediates adhesion between hematolymphoid cells and stromal cells has been identified (Kina *et al.*, 1991; Miyake *et al.*, 1991). It is tempting to speculate that this 107 kDa glycoprotein might be similar or identical to VCAM-1. It is expected that LPAM-2 ($\alpha_{4m}\beta_1$) binds to the mouse homologue of VCAM-1. However, the identity of the ligand(s) for LPAM-1 ($\alpha_{4m}\beta_p$) are still unknown. The availability of α_{4m} and β_p cDNAs may aid in the search for their ligand(s) on HEV in mucosal lymphoid organs.

VII. Concluding Perspective

Our knowledge of lymphocyte traffic in the body has progressed remarkably in the last 10 years, primarily because of the identification and characterization of a number of organ specific lymphocyte homing receptors, vascular addressins on HEV, and other cell adhesion molecules. The different ligand specificity, divalent cation requirements, and structure of these receptors and adhesion molecules suggest that each molecule contributes in a unique fashion to confer the final tissue specific adhesive interaction. The dynamic role of lymphocyte homing receptors in deploying the immunocompetent lymphocytes in lymphoid or nonlymphoid organs is not only engaged in targeting and anchoring functions but also may be involved in signaling pathways that transduce information from the particular extracellular environment to the interior of lymphocytes, influencing their proliferation and physiology. Searching for new lymphocyte homing receptors and their complementary ligands on HEV in lymphoid organs or tissues in nonlymphoid organs, studying structure function relationships of these receptors and interactions with the cytoskeleton, and signaling pathways will provide exciting insights into the mechanisms governing the control of lymphocyte traffic. The use of soluble forms of these receptors to investigate, and perhaps to control various inflammatory disease and tumor metastasis processes will be exploited. Further advances in our understanding of the mechanisms that direct lymphocyte migration will be very useful from both a scientific and clinical perspective.

Acknowledgments

We thank Lily Hu and Libuse Jerabek for their assistance with cell cultures and mouse work, respectively. This work was supported by the Howard Hughes Medical Institute and in part by National Institutes of Health Grants AI09072 and CA42551. M.H. is a postdoctoral fellow of the Leukemia Society of America and I.W. is an Investigator of the Howard Hughes Medical Institute.

References

Appella, E., Robinson, E. A., Ullrich, S. J., Stoppelli, M. P., Corti, A., Cassani, G., and Blasi, F. (1987). *J. Biol. Chem.* **262,** 4437–4440.

Argraves, W. S., Dickerson, K., Burgess, W. H., and Ruoslahti, E. (1989). *Cell* **58,** 623–629.

Argraves, W. S., Suzuki, S., Arai, H., Thompson, K., Pierschbacher, M. D., and Ruoslahti, E. (1987). *J. Cell. Biol.* **105,** 1183–1190.

Beer, J., and Coller, B. D. (1989). *J. Biol. Chem.* **264,** 17564–17573.

Buck, C. A., Shea, E., Duggan, K., and Horwitz, A. F. (1986). *J. Cell. Biol.* **103,** 2421–2428.

Burridge, K., Fath, K., Kelly, T., Nuckolis, B., and Turner, C. (1988). *Annu. Rev. Cell. Bio.* **4,** 487–525.

Butcher, E. C., Scollay, R. G., and Weissman, I. L. (1979). *J. Immunol.* **123,** 1996–2003.

Buyon, J. P., Slade, S. G., Reibman, J., Abramson, S. B., Philips, M. R., Weissmann, G., and Winchester, R. (1990). *J. Immunol.* **144,** 191–197.

Carpenter, G., and Cohen, S. (1979). *Ann. Rev. Biochem.* **48,** 193–216.

Carter, W. G., and Wayner, E. A. (1988). *J. Biol. Chem.* **263,** 4193–4201.

Chen, W-J., Goldstein, J. L., and Brown, M. S. (1990). *J. Biol. Chem.* **265,** 3116–3123.

Cheresh, D. A., Smith, J. W., Cooper, H. M., and Quaranta, V. (1989). *Cell* **57,** 59–69.

Cooke, R. M., Wilkinson, A. J., Baron, M., Pastore, A., Tappin, M. J., Campbell, I. D., Gregory, H., and Sheard, B. (1987). *Nature (London)* **327,** 339–341.

Davis, C. G., Goldstein, J. L., Sudhof, T. C., Anderson, R. G., Russell, D. W., and Brown, M. S. (1987). *Nature (London)* **326,** 760–765.

Davis, L. S., Oppenheimer-Marks, N., Bednarczyk, J. L., McIntyre, B. W., and Lipsky, P. E. (1990). *J. Immunol.* **145,** 785–793.

DeSimone, D., and Hynes, R. O. (1988). *J. Biol. Chem.* **263,** 5333–5340.

Devereux, I., Haeberli, P., and Smithies, O. (1984). *Nucl. Acids Res.* **12,** 387–395.

D'Souza, S. E., Ginsberg, M. H., Burke, T. A., Lam, S. C.-T., and Plow, E. F. (1988). *Science* **242,** 91–93.

Elices, M. J., Osborn, L., Takada, Y., Crouse, C., Luhowskyl, S., Hemler, M., and Lobb, R. (1990). *Cell* **60,** 577–584.

Freed, E., Gailit, J., van der Geer, P., Ruoslahti, E., and Hunter, T. (1989). *EMBO J.* **8,** 2955–2965.

Gallatin, M., St. John, T. P., Siegelman, M., Reichert, R., Butcher, E. C., and Weissman, I. L. (1986). *Cell* **44,** 673–680.

Garcia-Pardo, A., Wayner, E. A., Carter, W. G., and Ferreira, O. C., Jr. (1990). *J. Immunol.* **144,** 3361–3366.

Goldstein, L. A., Zhou, D. F. H., Picker, L. J., Minty, C. N., Bargatze, R. F., Ding, J. F., and Butcher, E. C. (1989). *Cell* **56,** 1063–1072.

Gowans, J., and Knight, E. (1964). *Phil. Trans. Roy. Soc. (London)* **B 159,** 257–282.

Graf, J., Iwamoto, Y., Sasaki, M., Martin, G. R., Kleinman, H. K., Robey, F. A., and Yamada, Y. (1987). *Cell* **48,** 989–996.

Gray, A., Dull, T., and Ullrich, A. (1983). *Nature (London)* **303,** 722–725.

Hamann, A., Jablonski-Westrich, D., Duijvenstijn, A., Butcher, E. C., Baisch, H., Harder, R., and Thiele, H. G. (1988). *J. Immunol.* **140,** 693–699.

Handford, P. A., Baron, M., Mayhew, M., Willis, A., Beesley, T., Brownlee, G. G., and Campbell, I. D. (1990). *EMBO J.* **9,** 475–480.

Heath, W. F., and Merrifield, R. B. (1986). *Proc. Natl. Acad. Sci. U.S.A.* **83,** 6367–6371.

Hemler, M. E. (1990). *Ann. Rev. Immunol.* **8,** 365–400.

Hemler, M. E., Crouse, C., and Sonnenberg, A. (1989). *J. Biol. Chem.* **264,** 6529–6535.

Hemler, M. E., Elices, M. J., Parker, C., and Takada, Y. (1990). *Immunol. Rev.* **114,** 45–65.

Hirst, R., Horwitz, A., Buck, C., and Rohrschneider, L. (1986). *Proc. Natl. Acad. Sci. U.S.A.* **83,** 6470–6474.

Hogervorst, F., Kuikman, I., von dem Borne, A. E. G. Jr., and Sonnenberg, A. (1990). *EMBO J.* **9,** 765–770.

Holers, V. M., Ruff, T. G., Parks, D. L., McDonald, J. A., Ballard, L. L., Brown, E. J. (1989). *J. Exp. Med.* **169,** 1589–1605.

Holzmann, B., McIntyre, B. W., and Weissman, I. L. (1989). *Cell* **56,** 37–46.

Holzmann, B., and Weissman, I. L. (1989a). *EMBO J.* **8,** 1735–1741.

Holzmann, B., and Weissman, I. L. (1989b). *Immunol. Rev.* **108,** 45–61.

Hunter, T., and Cooper, J. A. (1985). *Ann. Rev. Biochem.* **54,** 897–930.

Hynes, R. O. (1987). *Cell* **48,** 549–554.

Idzerda, R. L., Carter, W. G., Nottenburg, C., Wayner, E. A., Gallatin, W. M., and St. John, T. (1989). *Proc. Natl. Acad. Sci. U.S.A.* **86,** 4659–4663.

Jalkanen, S., Bargatze, R. F., Herron, L. R., and Butcher, E. C. (1986). *Eur. J. Immunol.* **16,** 1195–1202.

Jalkanen, S., Bargatze, R. F., de los Toyos, J., and Butcher, E. C. (1987). *J. Cell. Biol.* **105,** 983–990.

Kajiji, S., Tamura, R. N., and Quaranta, V. (1989). *EMBO J.* **8,** 673–680.

Kansas, G. S., Wood, G. S., and Dailey, M. O. (1989). *J. Immunol.* **142,** 3050–3057.

Kina, T., Majumdar, A. S., Heimfeld, S., Kaneshima, H., Holzmann, B., Katsura, Y., and Weissman, I. L. (1991). *J. Exp. Med.* **173,** 373–381.

Kishimoto, T. K., Larson, R. S., Corbi, A. L., Dustin, M. L., Staunton, D. E., and Springer, T. A. (1989). *Adv. Immunol.* **46,** 149–182.

Komoriya, A., Hortsch, M., Meyers, C., Smith, M., Kanety, H., and Schlessinger, J. (1984). *Proc. Natl. Acad. Sci. U.S.A.* **81,** 1351–1355.

Kurosawa, S., Stearns, D., Jackson, K., and Esmon, C. (1988). *J. Biol. Chem.* **263,** 5993–5996.

Larson, R. S., and Springer, T. A. (1990). *Immunol. Rev.* **114,** 181–217.

Lasky, L. A., Singer, M. S., Yednock, T. A., Dowbenko, D., Fennie, C., Rodriguez, H., Nguyen, T., Stachel, S., and Rosen, S. D. (1989). *Cell* **56,** 1045–1055.

Loftus, J. C., O'Toole, T. E., Plow, E. F., Glass, A., Frelinger III, A. L., and Ginsberg, M. H. (1990). *Science* **249,** 915–918.

MacKrell, A. J., Blumberg, B., Haynes, S. R., and Fessler, J. H. (1988). *Proc. Natl. Acad. Sci. U.S.A.* **85,** 2633–2637.

Miyake, K., Weissman, I. L., Greenberger, J. S., and Kincade, P. W. (1991). *J. Exp. Med.* **173,** 599–607.

Nermut, M. V., Green, N. M., Eason, P., Yamada, S. S., and Yamada, K. M. (1988). *EMBO J.* **7,** 4093–4099.

Neuhaus, H., Hu, M. C-T., Hemler, M. E., Yoshikazu, T., Holzmann, B., and Weissman, I. L. (1991). *J. Cell Biol.* (in press).

Nojima, Y., Humphries, M. J., Paul Mould, A., Komoriya, A., Yamada, K. M., Fchlossman, S. F., and Morimoto, C. (1990). *J. Exp. Med.* **172,** 1185–1192.

Osborn, L., Hession, C., Tizard, R., Vassallo, C., Luhowskyj, S., Chi-Rosso, G., and Lobb, R. (1989). *Cell* **59,** 1203–1211.

Pals, S. T., den Otter, A., Miedema, F., Kabel, P., Keizer, G. D., Schepper, R. J., and Meijer, C. J. L. M. (1988). *J. Immunol.* **140,** 1851–1853.

Phillips, D. R., Charo, I. F., Parise, L. V., and Fitzgerald, L. A. (1988). *Blood* **71,** 831–843.

Picker, L. J., de los Toyos, J., Telen, M. J., Haynes, B. F., and Butcher, E. C. (1989). *J. Immunol.* **142,** 2046–2051.

Ramaswamy, H., and Hemler, M. E. (1990). *EMBO J.* **9,** 1561–1568.

Rice, E. G., and Bevilacqua, M. (1989). *Science* **246,** 1303–1306.

Ruoslahti, E., and Giancotti, F. G. (1989). *Cancer Cells* **1,** 119–126.

Ruoslahti, E., and Pierschbacher, M. D. (1987). *Science* **238,** 491–497.

Scott, J., Urdea, M., Quiroga, M., Sanchez-Pescador, R., Fong, N., Selby, M., Rutter, W., and Bell, G. I. (1983). *Science* **221,** 236–240.

Sheppard, D., Rozzo, C., Starr, L., Quaranta, V., Erle, D. J., and Pytela, R. (1990). *J. Biol. Chem.* **265,** 11502–11507.

Siegelman, M. H., Cheng, I. C., Weissman, I. L., and Wakeland, E. K. (1990). *Cell* **61,** 611–622.

Siegelman, M. H., van de Rijn, M., and Weissman, I. L. (1989). *Science* **243,** 1165–1172.

Siegelman, M. H., and Weissman, I. L. (1989). *Proc. Natl. Acad. Sci. U.S.A.* **86,** 5562–5566.

Smith, J. W., and Cheresh, D. A. (1988). *J. Biol. Chem.* **263,** 18726–18731.

Solowska, J., Guan, J.-L., Marcantonio, E. E., Trevithick, J. E., Buck, C. A., and Hynes, R. O. (1989). *J. Cell. Biol.* **109,** 853–861.

Springer, T. A. (1990). *Nature (London).* **346,** 425–434.

Stamper, H. B., Jr., and Woodruff, J. J. (1976). *J. Exp. Med.* **144,** 828–833.

Stoolman, L. M. (1989). *Cell* **56,** 907–910.

Stoppelli, M. P., Corti, A., Soffientini, A., Cassani, G., Blasi, F., and Assoian, R. K. (1985). *Proc. Natl. Acad. Sci. U.S.A.* **82,** 4939–4943.

Streeter, P. R., Berg, E. L., Rouse, B. T. N., Bargatze, R. F., and Butcher, E. C. (1988a). *Nature (London)* **331,** 41–46.

Streeter, P. R., Rouse, B. T. N., and Butcher, E. C. (1988b). *J. Cell. Biol.* **107,** 1853–1862.

Strynadka, N., and James, M. (1989). *Annu. Rev. Biochem.* **58,** 951–998.

Suzuki, S., and Naitoh, Y. (1990). *EMBO J.* **9,** 757–763.

Takada, Y., Elices, M. J., Crouse, C., and Hemler, M. E. (1989). *EMBO J.* **8,** 1361–1368.

Tamkun, J. W., DeSimone, D. W., Fonda, D., Patel, R. S., Buck, C., Horwitz, A. F., and Hynes, R. O. (1986). *Cell* **46,** 271–282.

Tedder, T. F., Isaacs, C. M., Ernst, T. J., Demetri, G. D., Adler, D. A., and Disteche, C. M. (1989). *J. Exp. Med.* **170,** 123–133.

Tominaga, S. (1988). *FEBS Lett.* **238,** 315–319.

Vyas, N. K., Vyas, M. N., and Quiocho, F. A. (1987). *Nature (London)* **327,** 635–638.

Wayner, E. A., Garcia-Pardo, A., Humphries, M. J., MacDonald, J. A., and Carter, W. G. (1989). *J. Cell. Biol.* **109,** 1321–1330.

Wolf, H., Modrow, S., Motz, M., Jameson, B., Hermann, G., and Fortsch, B. (1987). *Computer Appl. in Biosci.* **4,** 187–191.

Yamamoto, T., Bishop, R. W., Brown, M. S., Goldstein, J. L., and Russell, D. W. (1986). *Science* **232,** 1230–1237.

CHAPTER 6

Vascular Addressins: Tissue Selective Endothelial Cell Adhesion Molecules for Lymphocyte Homing

Ellen L. Berg

Laboratory of Immunology and Vascular Biology
Department of Pathology
Stanford University, Stanford, California 94305 and the Center for Molecular Biology and Medicine, Veterans Administration Medical Center
Palo Alto, California 94304

Louis J. Picker

Department of Pathology
The University of Texas Southwestern Medical Center
Dallas, Texas 75235

Martyn K. Robinson

Celltech Ltd.
Slough SL14EN, England

Philip R. Streeter

SyStemix, Inc.
Palo Alto, California 94303

Eugene C. Butcher

Laboratory of Immunology and Vascular Biology
Department of Pathology, Stanford University
Stanford, California 94305 and the Center for Molecular Biology and Medicine, Veterans Administration Medical Center
Palo Alto, California 94304

I. Introduction

The adhesion of blood borne leukocytes to endothelial cells is the initial event in the process of lymphocyte entrance into lymphoid organs, and it is also one of the initial events in leukocyte recruitment into tissues at sites of inflammation. Lymphocytes are unique among the leukocytes in that they continuously traffic between the blood and lymphatic systems, entering lymphoid organs by first adhering to specialized high-walled post-capillary venules, known as high endothelial venules (HEV) (Gowans and Knight, 1964; Marchesi and Gowans, 1964) (Fig. 1). They exit lymph nodes through efferent lymphatics and pass back into the blood via the thoracic duct. HEV are found preferentially in lymphoid organs and in sites of chronic inflammation. Antigen specific lymphocyte responses are usually initiated in the lymphoid organs, and thus, the generation of memory responses are dependent on entrance of lymphocytes into these tissues. The effector functions of lymphocytes, as well as the leukocytes that compose the antigen nonspecific arm of the immune system, depend on their timely recruitment from the blood into tissues at sites of inflammation, the first step of which is also adhesion to vascular endothelium (reviewed in Carlos and Harlan, 1990). Indeed, the vascular endothelium at sites of inflammation can be modified by the inflammatory response so as to be more adhesive for specific leukocyte subsets (Jutila *et al.*, 1989a; Butcher, 1990; Cotran *et al.*, 1986; Munro *et al.*, 1989; Dustin *et al.*, 1986) (See Section III.B.3.). In both lymphoid organs and in sites of inflammation, specific receptor–ligand pairs between the leukocyte and endothelial cell mediate the adhesion process and thus control, in part, the type of cell that is to be recruited into the tissue parenchyma. For the trafficking of lymphocytes through lymph nodes and sites of chronic inflammation these molecules have been called *lymphocyte homing receptors* (Gallatin *et al.*, 1983) and *vascular addressins* (Streeter *et al.*, 1988a).

Lymphocyte interactions with HEV are characteristically tissue specific. Lymphocytes have the capacity to distinguish between HEV in peripheral lymph nodes, mucosal lymphoid tissues, the chronically inflamed synovium of arthritic joints, and chronically inflamed skin (see Section II). This capacity is controlled, in part, by the expression of distinct tissue specific homing receptors that recognize and bind to HEV ligands, the vascular addressins, which are selectively expressed in different lymphoid organs or chronically inflamed tissues (See Section III). Other leukocytes (for example, neutrophils, monocytes, etc.) can also express homing receptors and can interact in some instances with vascular addressins. The selectivity of neutrophil versus monocyte or lymphocyte recruitment during different

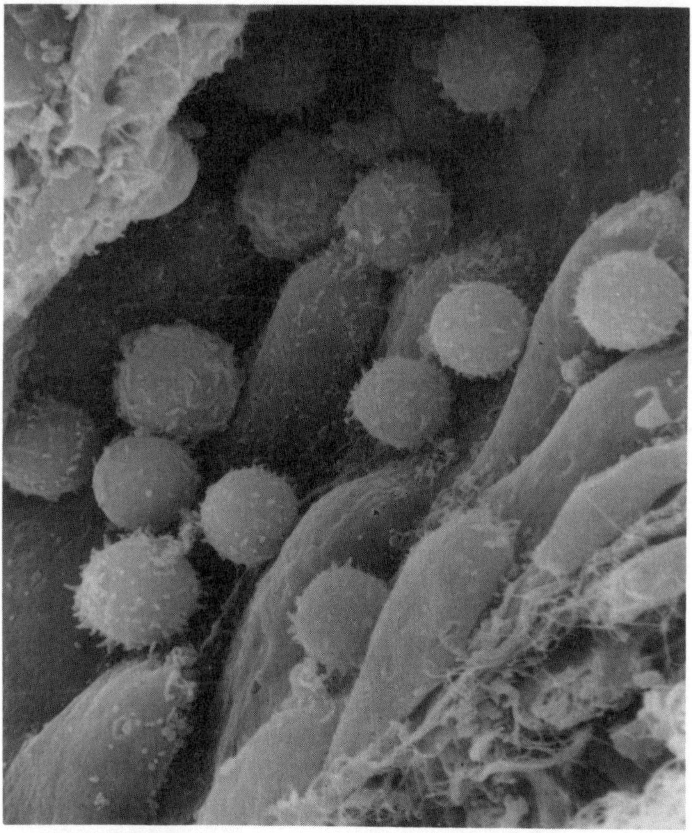

FIGURE 1

Scanning electron micrograph of the cut surface of a mouse lymph node showing numerous lymphocytes tightly bound to the plump endothelial cells of an HEV. Nonadherent blood elements were washed out by flushing the vasculature with medium prior to fixation by perfusion with glutaraldehyde. (Reprinted with permission from Butcher *et al.*, 1982).

states of inflammation is likely governed by the expression and activation states of multiple leukocyte cell adhesion molecules, including but not limited to tissue specific homing receptors and their endothelial cell ligands.

II. Lymphocyte Interactions with High Endothelial Venules

Lymphocyte interactions with HEV were first modeled *in vitro* by Stamper and Woodruff (1976). In this assay, lymphocytes bind specifically to the HEV within frozen sections of lymphoid tissues (Fig. 2). The ability of different lymphocyte populations to bind HEV parallels faithfully lymphocyte–HEV interactions *in vivo* (Butcher *et al.*, 1979a). Lymphocytes are also able to distinguish between HEV in different lymphoid organs in this assay (Butcher *et al.*, 1980; Jalkanen *et al.*, 1986a). Distinct recognition systems have been demonstrated for peripheral lymph nodes (PLN), mucosal lymphoid organs such as the Peyer's patches (PP) and appendix, and the synovium of chronically inflamed joints (Butcher *et al.*, 1980; Jalkanen *et al.*, 1986b). Other studies indicate that additional lymphocyte–HEV recognition systems may control lymphocyte entrance into peribronchial lymph nodes, pulmonary lymphoid aggregates (Geoffroy *et al.*, 1988), and chronically inflamed skin (Chin *et al.*, 1988; Picker *et al.*, 1991). Lymphocyte receptors that confer tissue specificity are known as *homing receptors* and their HEV counterreceptors as *vascular addressins*.

The ability of lymphocytes to adhere to particular HEV is regulated during development as well as during antigen driven differentiation. Nonrecirculating lymphocytes, such as germinal center B-cells and cortical thymocytes, do not adhere to HEV *in vitro* while most naive recirculating lymphocytes (mature cells that have not yet encountered antigen) express homing receptors allowing their traffic to lymph nodes, Peyer's patches, and spleen (Butcher *et al.*, 1979a; Scollay *et al.*, 1980; Reichert *et al.*, 1983). Among these "virgin" cells, the predominance of B-cells in PP and T-cells in PLN reflects in part the quantitative difference in the adhesiveness of these cells for the HEV in PP and PLN, respectively (Stevens *et al.*, 1982). However, subsets of effector and memory cells display more dramatic restrictions in HEV binding capacities and homing receptor expression, which reflect the site in which they first encounter antigen (reviewed in Butcher, 1986) (See Section III.B.).

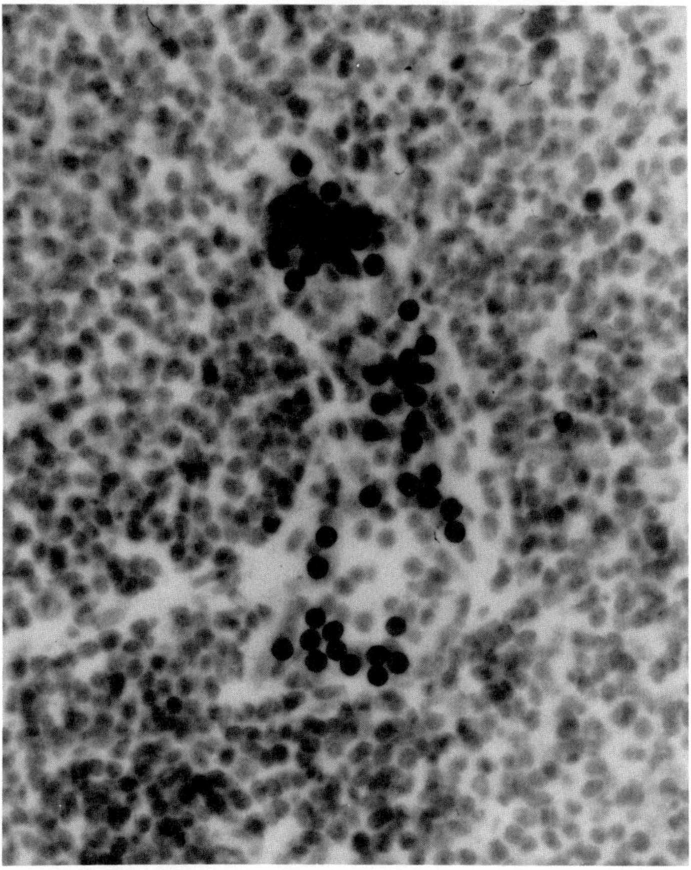

FIGURE 2

Selective binding of lymphocytes to an HEV in a frozen section of a mouse lymph node. Lymphocytes were incubated at 7°C for 30 minutes on fresh frozen sections of a mouse lymph node and cells bound to HEV were fixed to the section with glutaraldehyde in PBS. Adherent cells were easily visualized because they stain more heavily with thionine than the underlying tissue. [Reprinted by permission from Butcher *et al.*, (1979b) *Nature* **280**, 497, Copyright © 1983 Macmillan Magazines Ltd.]

III. Molecules Involved in Tissue-Specific Lymphocyte Interactions with Endothelial Cells

A. Vascular Addressins

Vascular addressins, tissue selective vascular adhesion molecules for lymphocytes, were named for their role in providing tissue position information or address signals to circulating lymphocytes (Streeter *et al.*, 1988a, b). Three vascular addressins for lymphocytes have now been identified, the *peripheral lymph node addressin* (PNAd), which is selectively expressed in PLN HEV; the *mucosal addressin* (MAd), which is expressed by HEV in mucosal lymphoid organs such as the Peyer's patches and appendix; and a *skin vascular addressin*, ELAM-1, which during chronic inflammation is expressed preferentially by venules in the skin and appears to regulate the traffic of a skin specific memory lymphocyte population to this site.

1. The Musocal Addressin

The MAd was identified in the mouse by monoclonal antibodies MECA-367 and MECA-89, which selectively recognize HEV within PP and mesenteric lymph nodes (MLN) but not HEV in PLN (Streeter, *et al.*, 1988a) (Fig. 3). MAd is also expressed by venules in the gut lamina propria and mammary gland, vessels that also support lymphocyte traffic of mucosa associated lymphoid populations, such as IgA plasma cell precursors. Occasional small vessels in the pancreas and a thin layer of cells lining the marginal sinus around splenic white pulp nodules in the spleen also express MAd (E. Berg and P. Streeter, personal observations). Although high endothelial cell morphology clearly correlates with an increased capacity to promote lymphocyte traffic, lymphocyte trafficking is not restricted to HEV and within mucosal tissues, the expression of mucosal addressin in flat walled venules of the lamina propria reflects this. Indeed, the expression of MAd throughout mucosa associated tissues allows physically separated mucosal surfaces to be served by a common mucosal immune system, characterized by dissemination of specialized mucosal effector cells to all mucosal sites (McDermott and Bienenstock, 1979; reviewed in Butcher, 1986).

MAd is not detectable on endothelium in nonmucosal sites of acute inflammation nor in cutaneous CFA induced chronic granulomas in the mouse (M. Jutila and E. Berg, personal observations). However, in lymphocytic infiltrates within the chronically inflamed pancreas of nonobese

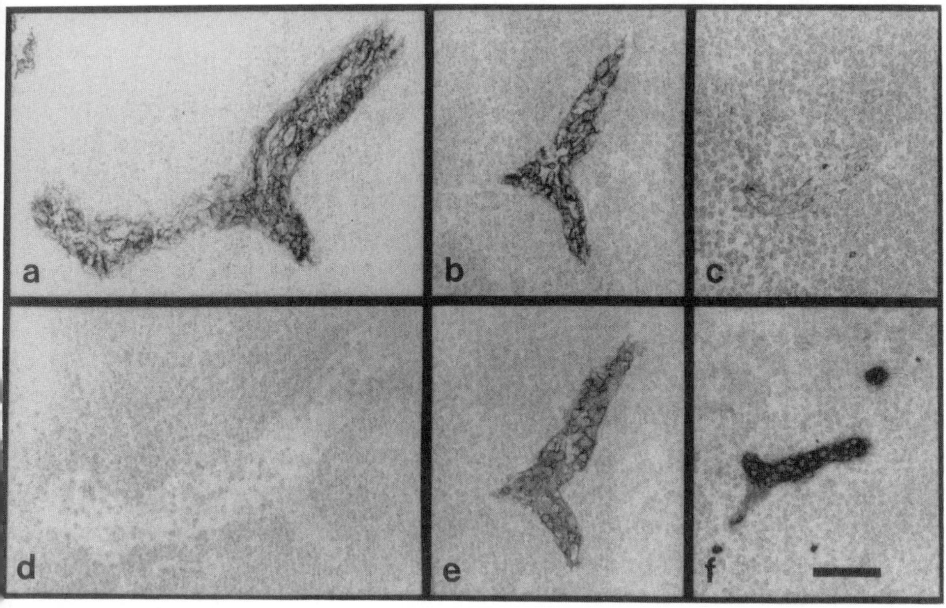

FIGURE 3

Analysis of PNAd (a–c) and MAd (d–f) on the lumenal surface of HEV in peripheral lymph nodes (PLN) (a and d), mesenteric lymph nodes (MLN) (b and e) and Peyer's patches (PP) (c and f). Monoclonal antibodies MECA-79 (rat IgM anti-PNAd) and MECA-367 (rat IgG_{2a} anti-MAd) were administered intravenously into mice and recipients sacrificed 15 minutes later. After perfusion to remove unbound antibody, lymphoid tissues were prepared for immunohistology. Serial sections were stained with the appropriate secondary antibodies coupled to peroxidase. Bar is 50μm. [Reproduced from Streeter *et al.* (1988b) *J. Cell Biol.* **107**, 1857, by copyright permission of the Rockefeller University Press.]

diabetic mice, many MECA-367 reactive vessels can be observed, some of these with the morphology of HEV (P. Streeter, unpublished data). In addition, some endothelial venules in the central nervous system express MAd during relapsing episodes of chronic experimental allergic encephalomyelitis but not during the initial or acute phases (O'Neill *et al.*, 1991).

In frozen section assays, MECA-367 blocks adhesion of lymphocytes to PP HEV almost completely but does not block binding to HEV in PLN (Streeter *et al.*, 1988a). The binding of lymphocytes to MLN is blocked 50%, which is consistent with MLN HEV having both mucosal and peripheral specificities. When injected *in vivo*, MECA-367 blocks the entry of transfused lymphocytes into PP completely and MLN partially, but does not block entry of lymphocytes into PLN. The extravasation of gut homing thoracic duct lymphoblasts into PP, MLN, or gut lamina propria, however, is only blocked 50% by MECA-367, suggesting that these cells may employ additional mechanisms for entrance into these tissues (P. Streeter and G. Griffiths, unpublished data).

MAd is a single chain glycoprotein of 58 to 66 kDa (Streeter *et al.*, 1988a). It contains sialic acid that appears to be O-linked as it is not sensitive to peptide N-glycosidase F (E. Berg, in preparation). Isolated MAd, incorporated into artificial planar lipid membranes, avidly binds lymphocytes and mucosal HEV binding cell lines (Nakache *et al.*, 1988). Binding of lymphocytes to MAd displays the same characteristics as does binding of lymphocytes to PP HEV, in that it is blocked by MECA-367; however, no antilymphocyte antibodies have yet been demonstrated to block adhesion of lymphocytes to the isolated MAd (See Section B.2.).

2. *The Peripheral Lymph Node Addressin*

Monoclonal antibody MECA-79 identifies the PNAd in both mouse and man (Streeter *et al.*, 1988b; 1991). In the mouse, MECA-79 stains all PLN HEV and many MLN HEV intensely, but in most mouse strains, it reacts only weakly with PP HEV (Fig. 3). Interestingly, in mouse strains that express increased levels of MECA-79 on PP HEV, these vessels have increased capacities to bind PLN–HEV specific cell lines and support entrance of these cells into PP in short-term *in vivo* homing experiments (Bargatze *et al.*, 1990). Lamina propria vessels in the gut, which express MAd, completely lack PNAd. In humans, MECA-79 reacts with HEV in PLN, tonsils, and some sites of extralymphoid chronic inflammation (Streeter *et al.*, 1991). Lamina propria vessels in the small intestine are negative, as in the mouse, but HEV in human mucosal lymphoid tissues (PP and appendix) stain with MECA-79, albeit less intensely than PLN HEV. In both mouse and man, MECA-79 inhibits lymphocyte binding to PLN HEV but not substantially to HEV in mouse PP or human appendix, in which binding via MAd appears to predominate. In short-term homing experiments in the mouse, MECA-79 blocks entrance of transfused lymphocytes into PLN but not into PP (Streeter *et al.*, 1988b).

MECA-79 recognizes a number of species with distinct molecular weights from PLN or tonsils lysates, although the most predominant by silver stain or Western blot is 105 kDa in the human and 90 and 115 kDa in the mouse (Berg *et al.*, 1991a, b). The MECA-79 epitope is likely conferred by posttranslational modification and may be carbohydrate in nature. The epitope is resistant to reduction and denaturation by treatments known to favor the preservation of carbohydrate determinants, although it is resistant to neuraminidase and peptide N-glycosidase F, which removes most N-linked sugars. A subset of mucosal addressin in the mouse MLN is decorated with the MECA-79 epitope, most obvious in MLN, in which many individual HEV cells express both PNAd and MAd (Fig. 3) (Streeter *et al.*, 1988b; Berg *et al.*, 1991b). These data indicate that the PNAd determinant can modify more than one glycoprotein, one of which can be the mucosal addressin.

In newborn mice, venules within PLN as well PP and MLN express MAd exclusively. PLN HEV from these animals are functionally mucosal as mucosal–HEV binding cell lines but not PLN–HEV specific cell lines bind to them in frozen sections. Only when mice are 1 to 2 weeks of age do venules within PLN begin to express PNAd, lose MAd expression, and begin to develop functional peripheral specificity (P. Streeter, unpublished data). Thus the development of peripheral specificity in PLN HEV involves both the induction of the PNAd determinant as well as the loss of MAd expression.

Immunoisolated PNAd from human tonsil is adhesive for lymphocytes. When coated on glass slides, only lymphocytes (Fig. 4) and PLN–HEV binding cell lines bind to PNAd. Mucosal HEV specific cell lines do not bind. The interaction is blocked by MECA-79 and also by antibodies against LECAM-1, the peripheral lymph node homing receptor (Berg *et al.*, 1991a) (See Section B.1.). In addition, an HEV nonbinding cell line, L1-2, when transfected with mouse LECAM-1 cDNA but not vector cDNA binds the isolated PNAd. That neuraminidase treatment of PNAd blocks lymphocyte attachment suggests involvement of sialic acid residues on PNAd in the interaction (See Section B.1.).

3. *ELAM-1 Is a Skin Vascular Addressin*

Endothelial-leukocyte adhesion molecule-1, ELAM-1, has been described as an inducible endothelial cell adhesion molecule for neutrophils (Bevilacqua *et al.*, 1987; Pober *et al.*, 1986). The 115 kDa ELAM-1 glycoprotein belongs to the LEC-CAM or SELECTIN gene family, which includes two other lectin adhesion molecules involved in inflammatory cell interactions, LECAM-1 (See Section B.1.) and GMP-140 (Bevilacqua *et al.*, 1989; Siegelman *et al.*, 1989; Lasky *et al.*, 1989; Tedder *et al.*, 1989; Camerini *et al.*, 1989; Kishimoto *et al.*, 1990; Johnston, *et al.*, 1989). The LEC-CAMs are characterized by an N-terminal domain homologous to C-type lectins,

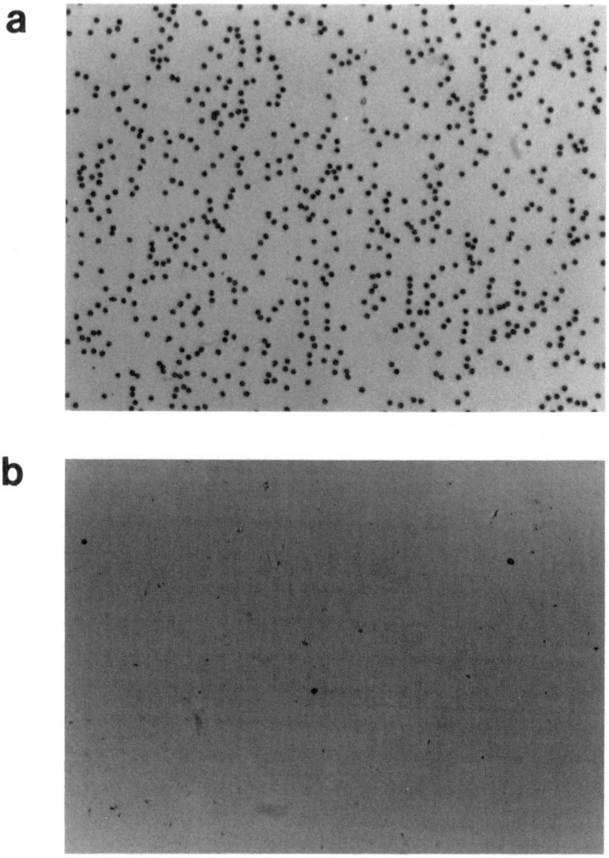

FIGURE 4

Lymphocytes bind avidly to immunoisolated peripheral lymph node addressin (PNAd). Samples of PNAd (a) or HCAM (b) isolated from human tonsil were absorbed onto glass slides. After blocking in serum containing medium, mouse PLN lymphocytes were applied to each and incubated at room temperature for 20 minutes under shear force. After washing and fixation with glutaraldehyde, bound cells were stained with thionine.

an EGF-like domain, a variable number of repeat sequences homologous to those found in complement regulatory proteins, a transmembrane domain, and a short cytoplasmic tail (reviewed in Stoolman, 1989). ELAM-1 is involved in the adhesion of neutrophils to cytokine activated human umbilical vein endothelial cells (HUVEC) *in vitro* and is rapidly induced on HUVEC by IL-1, TNF-alpha, and LPS and is also upregulated on a subset of venules in sites of acute inflammation *in vivo* (Cotran *et al.*, 1986; Munro *et al.*, 1989; Bevilacqua *et al.*, 1987; Pober *et al.*, 1986). However, an immunohistologic survey of chronically inflamed tissue specimens revealed intense ELAM-1 expression on venules in settings dominated by mononuclear cell influx. Furthermore, the expression of ELAM-1 was highly selective for skin sites of chronic inflammation (Picker *et al.*, 1991). Although ELAM-1 was found on venules in some extracutaneous sites of chronic inflammation, the degree of expression was substantially less than that observed in the majority of skin lesions. Interestingly, COS cells transfected with ELAM-1 cDNA not only bind neutrophils but also selectively bind a unique skin associated population of T-cells of memory phenotype, characterized by the expression of a cutaneous lymphocyte associated antigen, CLA, which is observed almost exclusively in cutaneous inflammatory sites and as a circulating memory T-cell subset in blood (Picker *et al.*, 1991; Picker *et al.*, 1990a, b) (See Section III.B.3.). Thus, ELAM-1 is a skin vascular addressin for these unique skin homing memory T-cells. These findings are consistent with earlier experiments indicating that lymphocyte binding to venules in chronically inflamed skin occurs via mechanisms distinct from those targeting lymphocytes to peripheral and mucosal lymphoid organs (Chin *et al.*, 1988; Sackstein *et al.*, 1988; Wu *et al.*, unpublished results). The paucity of CLA^+ lymphocytes in inflamed synovia, in combination with the expression of only low levels of ELAM-1 in association with lymphoid aggregates in this setting, suggests that homing to synovium and to the skin is also differentially regulated (Picker *et al.*, 1991).

B. Homing Receptors

Quite a number of lymphocyte molecules have been implicated in HEV binding, as evidenced by the ability of specific antibodies to inhibit the interaction of lymphocytes with HEV. The molecules involved in tissue specific endothelial cell recognition have been called homing receptors. Here we consider these particularly in the context of their interaction with the known vascular addressins (Table I).

TABLE I

Endothelial Cell Vascular Addressins and Their Known Lymphocyte Ligands in Mouse and Man

Tissue	Vascular addressin	Lymphocyte homing receptor
Peripheral lymph nodes	PNAd	LECAM-1
Mucosal lymphoid organs (PP, MLN, appendix, etc.)	MAd ? ?	? LPAM-1 HCAM (CD44)
Chronically inflamed skin	ELAM-1	CLA?

1. LECAM-1, the Peripheral Lymph Node Homing Receptor

The peripheral lymph node homing receptor, now known as LECAM-1, was first identified in the mouse by monoclonal antibody MEL-14 (Gallatin *et al.*, 1983). MEL-14 blocks lymphocyte binding to PLN HEV but not PP HEV and selectively recognizes PLN HEV binding cell lines. *In vivo*, MEL-14 selectively stains lymphocytes capable of recirculating. Most thymocytes and germinal center B-cells, normally sessile populations, are MEL-14^-. The molecular cloning of LECAM-1 (the MEL-14 or Ly-22 antigens in the mouse, and Dreg-56, Leu-8, LAM-1 or TQ1 antigens in the human) has revealed its homology with the LEC-CAM or SELECTIN gene family (Siegelman *et al.*, 1989; Lasky *et al.*, 1989; Tedder *et al.*, 1989; Stoolman, 1989). The relationship of LECAM-1 to the rat PLN homing receptor, $HEBF_{LN}$, identified by the A.11 monoclonal antibody (Rasmussen *et al.*, 1985) is not yet known. LECAM-1 is a highly glycosylated protein of approximately 70 to 90 kDa with a core peptide of 42 kDa. Studies confirm that LECAM-1 indeed appears to function as a calcium dependent carbohydrate binding molecule (Imai *et al.*, 1990). Many years previous to the molecular cloning of LECAM-1, carbohydrate determinants had been implicated in lymphocyte adhesion to PLN HEV (Stoolman *et al.*, 1984; Rosen *et al.*, 1985; Yednock *et al.*, 1987). A number of anionic mono- and polysaccharides blocked lymphocyte attachment to PLN HEV including mannose-6-phosphate, fructose-1-phosphate, fucoidan, a highly sulfated and fucosylated polysaccharide, and the mannose-6-phosphate rich yeast mannan PPME, albeit at high concentrations. It was also found that neuraminidase treatment of frozen sections of lymphoid organs blocks binding of lymphocytes to PLN but not to PP HEV (Rosen *et al.*, 1985). The ability of

LECAM-1 cDNA transfectants to bind to isolated peripheral lymph node addressin, PNAd, as described earlier, has also confirmed the role of carbohydrate moieties in LECAM-1–ligand interactions. Binding of cells, via LECAM-1, to PNAd is dependent on calcium and sensitive to neuraminidase treatment of PNAd (Berg *et al.*, 1991a).

The pattern of LECAM-1 expression on lymphocytes supports the observation that lymphocytes become restricted in their trafficking patterns following antigen driven maturation. In the human, among mature T-cells (cells that are $CD3^{hi}$ and either $CD8^{+}$ or $CD4^{+}$), previously activated T-cells (enriched for memory for recall antigens) can be distinguished from presumed virgin T-cells by their higher expression of several adhesion molecules especially LFA-3 (Sanders *et al.*, 1988) and also their preferential expression of CD45RO over CD45RA (Akbar *et al.*, 1988). While virgin T-cells express LECAM-1 at a uniformly high level, only a portion of memory T-cells express LECAM-1 (Picker *et al.*, 1990b). Interestingly, the level of LECAM-1 expression by these memory T-cells is slightly higher than that by virgin T-cells. Mucosal associated effector lymphocyte populations, however, do not express LECAM-1. Mucosal associated memory T-cells found preferentially in the gut epithelium and lamina propria and identified by expression of the mucosal lymphocyte antigen (MLA), defined by monoclonal antibodies HML-1 and Ber ACT8 (Cerf-Bensussan *et al.*, 1987; Kruschwitz *et al.*, 1991), do not express LECAM-1 (Schieferdecker *et al.*, 1990). MLA^{+} cells in the blood, presumably gut homing cells, also uniformly lack LECAM-1 (Picker *et al.*, 1990b). In the mouse, gut intraepithelial cells, which bind well to PP HEV but not to PLN HEV, have also been demonstrated to lack LECAM-1 (Schmitz *et al.*, 1988). These data indicate that the expression of homing receptors on lymphocytes is indeed selective among memory cells and that restricted patterns of homing receptor expression may be a diagnostic feature of memory cells.

LECAM-1 is expressed by neutrophils, monocytes, and other leukocytes as well as lymphocytes, although these cells do not normally traffic through HEV (Lewinsohn *et al.*, 1987; Jutila *et al.*, 1989b). Interaction of neutrophil or monocyte LECAM-1 with PNAd in the absence of additional inflammation induced adhesion molecules or inflammation associated activation signals, may be insufficient to promote adhesion, emigration, or both through HEV. Interestingly, monocytes, unlike lymphocytes, do not bind to immunoisolated PNAd (E. Berg, personal observations). In frozen sections, monocytes bind only to PLN HEV from inflamed lymph nodes. This adhesion is blocked by both anti-LECAM-1 antibody as well as by antibodies against Mac-1 (Jutila *et al.*, 1989a; 1990). This suggests that while LECAM-1 interaction with PNAd alone is insufficient to promote monocyte trafficking through PLN HEV, it may participate in trafficking of monocytes through inflamed PLN HEV in the presence of additional adhesive mechanisms.

Neutrophil LECAM-1 has been shown to be involved in the recruitment of neutrophils to sites of acute inflammation (Jutila *et al.*, 1989b; 1990), sites in which PNAd is not expressed (E. Berg and M. Jutila, personal observations). Chemotactic factor stimulation of neutrophils results in their loss of surface LECAM-1 with a concomitant increase in Mac-1 expression (Jutila *et al.*, 1989a,b; Kishimoto *et al.*, 1989; 1990). In addition, these cells no longer have the capacity to traffic to inflammatory sites. Although there appears to be just one gene for LECAM-1 (Ord *et al.*, 1990), the neutrophil and monocyte forms are larger than lymphocyte LECAM-1 (105 and 130 kDa versus the 90 kDa lymphocyte form) (Lewinsohn *et al.*, 1987; Jutila *et al.*, 1990). Thus the ligands for each of these may, in some cases, be distinct and may not necessarily function via the calcium dependent lectin domain of LECAM-1.

2. *Mucosal Homing Receptor(s)*

The mucosal or gut associated lymphoid tissues include the PP, MLN, gut epithelium, and lamina propria (McDermott and Bienenstock, 1979). This system involves the trafficking of lymphocytes through these tissues as well as the spleen. At least one vascular addressin, MAd, has been identified that is specifically expressed on HEV and EC in these tissues (See Section A.2.) and is an adhesion molecule for mucosal homing lymphocytes (Streeter *et al.*, 1988a; Nakache *et al.*, 1988). However, the lymphocyte ligand for this molecule has not yet been identified.

Several lymphocyte surface molecules have been proposed as mucosal homing receptors based on the ability of monoclonal antibodies to specifically block binding of lymphocytes to PP HEV but not PLN HEV in frozen sections. MAb Hermes-3 against HCAM (the Hermes antigen, CD44) blocks human lymphocytes from binding to PP but not to PLN or synovial HEV (Jalkanen *et al.*, 1987). However, HCAM is expressed by a wide variety of cell types and not just leukocytes (Picker *et al.*, 1989). Furthermore, it is not heterogeneously expressed on memory T-cells, which instead uniformly express HCAM at a level higher than that found on virgin T-cells (Picker *et al.*, 1990b). Although HCAM purified from diverse cell types has been shown by energy transfer measurements to interact with isolated MAd (Picker *et al.*, 1989; M. Nakache, unpublished results), HCAM has also been demonstrated to interact with a variety of ligands, including fibronectin, collagen type IV, and hyaluronic acid (Carter and Wayner, 1988; Culty *et al.*, 1990; S. Jalkanen, in preparation).

Together these data suggest that HCAM may function as an important accessory molecule for HEV binding but may not be the tissue specific element responsible for initial recognition of MAd.

Another proposed mucosal homing receptor is LPAM-1 (Holzmann *et al.*, 1989). LPAM-1 ($\alpha_4\beta_p$) belongs to the integrin gene family and is related to VLA-4 ($\alpha_4\beta_1$). Monoclonal antibody R1/2 selectively blocks mouse lymphocytes from binding to PP HEV. Monoclonal antibodies against α_4 in the human also block lymphocyte binding to PP or appendix HEV (Holtzmann *et al.*, unpublished results). An analysis of the expression pattern of LPAM-1 is complicated by the fact that antibodies to β_p, the unique β chain of LPAM-1, are not yet reported. Nevertheless, MLA^+ cells are $\alpha_4{}^{hi}$ and $\beta_1{}^{lo}$, raising the possibility that gut associated T-cells express $\alpha_4\beta_p$ selectively (Picker *et al.*, 1990b). Whether or not these cells are preferentially $\beta_p{}^{hi}$ remains to be determined. Several ligands for $\alpha_4\beta_1$ have been identified including fibronectin and VCAM-1, an inducible endothelial cell antigen found in some sites of chronic inflammation *in vivo* and on dendritic cells in a variety of lymphoid tissues (Wayner *et al.*, 1989; Guan and Hynes, 1990; Elices *et al.*, 1990). It is not known whether or not LPAM-1 can also interact with these ligands.

LPAM-1 does not appear to be a receptor for MAd. The monoclonal antibody R1/2 does not block lymphocyte binding to the isolated addressin (E. Berg, unpublished results). It may be that LPAM-1 has an alternative PP HEV ligand, or like HCAM, it may function as an accessory molecule but not a tissue specific restricting element for PP HEV. Although the human or mouse homologues of the rat mucosal homing receptor, $HEBF_{PP}$ (Chin *et al.*, 1986), have not yet been identified, this 80 kDa molecule may function as a ligand for MAd. It is likely that a number of homing receptors and their endothelial cell ligands are involved in trafficking through mucosal associated lymphoid tissues. The expression of MAd by PP and MLN HEV, lamina propria venules, and spleen, however, argues that it may be a major endothelial cell addressin unifying diverse mucosal tissues.

3. Cutaneous Lymphocyte Antigen, CLA, a Skin Homing Receptor?

The cutaneous lymphocyte antigen, CLA, is a carbohydrate antigen recognized by monoclonal antibody HECA-452 that is preferentially expressed on T-cells in cutaneous inflammatory lesions and on nearly all cutaneous intraepithelial T-cells (Picker *et al.*, 1990a). Its expression on blood T-lymphocytes is restricted to a subset of memory cells that do not include the MLA^+ subset (Picker *et al.*, 1990b). Blood CLA^+ cells are largely

LECAM-1^{hi} in most but not all samples; this may reflect the intimate association of the skin and its draining PLN, which are collectively referred to as skin associated lymphoid tissues or SALT (Streilein, 1983).

As described in Section A.3., CLA$^+$ lymphocytes bind selectively and avidly to ELAM-1. As ELAM-1 is expressed as a cutaneous vascular addressin in chronically inflamed skin, the specificity of ELAM-1 for CLA$^+$lymphocytes raised the possibility that CLA is a ligand for ELAM-1 and thus a skin homing receptor.

Sialated Lewis X antigen (sLe^x) has been identified as a major ELAM-1 ligand on neutrophils (Lowe *et al.*, 1990; Phillips *et al.*, 1990; Walz *et al.*, 1990) and indeed neutrophil sLe^x appears to be recognized by mAb HECA-452 (L. Rott, T. Yoshino, E. Berg, personal observations). However, lymphocytes, including CLA$^+$ lymphocytes, do not express significant levels of sLe^x (Ohmori *et al.*, 1989; L. Rott and E. Berg, personal observations). The HECA-452 Ag is expressed by a variety of cell types including lymphocytes, neutrophils, monocytes, HEV, and tonsil epithelium (Duijvestijn *et al.*, 1988; Picker *et al.*, 1990a). Interestingly, all of these cell types (only some of which express sLe^x) specifically bind ELAM-1 cDNA transfectants. HECA-452 immunoisolates from tonsil or monomyelomonocytic cell lines do bind ELAM-1 transfectants, suggesting that most or all HECA-452 reactive structures are ligands for ELAM-1 and that on neutrophils, but not on CLA$^+$ lymphocytes, this structure includes sLe^x. Indeed, the specificity of HECA-452 for carbohydrate structures in man appears to resemble closely the specificity of ELAM-1. It is likely that CLA itself on lymphocytes is a skin homing receptor for ELAM-1 in cutaneous chronic inflammation.

Acknowledgments

This work was supported in part by NIH grants GM37734, GM41965, AI19957, and DK38707 and by awards from the American Cancer Society and the Veterans Administration. E. Berg is a special fellow of the Leukemia Society of American, and E. Butcher is an Established Investigator of the American Heart Association.

References

Akbar, A. N., Terr, L., Timms, A., Beverly, P. C. L., and Janossy, G. (1988). *J. Immunol.* **140**, 2171–2178.

Bargatze, R. F., Streeter, P. R., and Butcher, E. C. (1990). *J. Cell. Biochem.* **42**, 219–227.
Berg, E. L., Robinson, M. K., Warnock, R. A., and Butcher, E. C. (1991a). *J. Cell Biol.* (in press).
Berg, E. L., Streeter, P. R., and Butcher, E. C. (1991b). Submitted for publication.
Bevilacqua, M. P., Pober, J. S., Mendrick, D. L., Cotran, R. S., and Gimbrone, M. A., Jr. (1987). *Proc. Natl. Acad. Sci. U.S.A.* **84**, 9238–9242.
Bevilacqua, M. P., Stengelin, S., Gimbrone, M. A., Jr., and Seed, B. (1989). *Science* **243**, 1160–1165.
Butcher, E. C. (1986). *Curr. Top. Micro. and Immunol.* **128**, 85–122.
Butcher, E. C. (1990). *Am. J. Pathol.* **136**, 3–11.
Butcher, E. C., Kraal, G., Stevens, S. K., and Weissman, I. L. (1982). *In* "Pathobiology of the Endothelial Cell" (H. L. Nossel and H. J. Vogel, eds.), p. 411. Academic Press, New York.
Butcher, E. C., Scollay, R. G., and Weissman, I. L. (1979a). *J. Immunol.* **123**, 1996–2003.
Butcher, E. C., Scollay, R. G., and Weissman, I. L. (1979b). *Nature (London)* **280**, 496–498.
Butcher, E. C., Scollay, R. G., and Weissman, I. L. (1980). *Eur. J. Immunol.* **10**, 556–561.
Camerini, D., James, S. P., Stamenkovic, I., and Seed, B. (1989). *Nature (London)* **342**, 78–82.
Carlos, T. M., and Harlan, J. M. (1990). *Imm. Rev.* **114**, 5–28.
Carter, W. G., and Wayner, E. A. (1988). *J. Biol. Chem.* **263**, 4193–4201.
Cerf-Bensussan, N., Jarry, A., Brousse, N., Lisowska-Grospierre, B., Guy-Grand, D., and Griscelli, C. (1987). *Eur. J. Immunol.* **17**, 1279–1285.
Chin, Y. H., Rasmussen, R. A., Woodruff, J. J., and Easton, T. G. (1986). *J. Immunol.* **136**, 2556–2561.
Chin, Y. H., Falanga, V., Streilein, J. W., and Sackstein, R. (1988). *Reg. Immunol.* **1**, 78–83.
Cotran, R. S., Gimbrone, M. A., Jr., Bevilacqua, M. P., Mendrick, D. L., and Pober, J. S. (1986). *J. Exp. Med.* **164**, 661–666.
Culty, M., Mayahe, K., Kincade, P. W., Sikorski, E., Butcher, E. C., and Underhill, C. (1990). *J. Cell. Biol.* **111**, 2765–2774.
Duijvestijn, A., Horst, E., Pals, S. T., Rouse, B. N., Steere, A. C., Picker, L. J., Meijer, C. J., and Butcher, E. C. (1988). *Am. J. Pathol.* **130**, 147–155.
Dustin, M. L., Rothlein, R., Bhan, A. K., Dinarello, C. D., and Springer, T. A. (1986). *J. Immunol.* **137**, 245–254.
Elices, M. J., Osborn, L., Takada, Y., Crouse, C., Luhowsky, S., Hemler, M. E., and Lobb, R. R. (1990). *Cell* **60**, 577–584.
Gallatin, W. M., Weissman, I. L., and Butcher, E. C. (1983). *Nature (London)* **304**, 30–34.
Geoffroy, J. S., Yednock, T. A., Curtis, J. L., and Rosen, S. D. (1988). *FASEB J.* **2**, A667.
Gowans, J. L., and Knight, E. J. (1964). *Proc. R. Soc. Lond. [Biol.]* **159**, 257–282.
Guan, J.-L., and Hynes, R. O. (1990). *Cell* **60**, 53–61.
Holzmann, B., McIntyre, B. W., and Weissman, I. L. (1989). *Cell* **56**, 37–46.
Imai, Y., True, D. D., Singer, M. S., and Rosen, S. D. (1990). *J. Cell. Biol.* **111**, 1225–1232.
Jalkanen, S. T., Bargatze, R. F., de los Toyos, J., and Butcher, E. C. (1986a). *J. Cell. Biol.* **105**, 983–990.
Jalkanen, S. T., Bargatze, R. F., de los Toyos, J., and Butcher, E. C. (1987). *J. Cell. Biol.* **105**, 983–990.
Jalkanen, S. T., Steere, A., Fox, R., and Butcher, E. C. (1986b). *Science* **233**, 556–558.
Johnston, G. I., Cook, R. G., and McEver, R. P. (1989). *Cell* **56**, 1033–1044.
Jutila, M. A., Berg, E. L., Kishimoto, T. K., Picker, L. J., Bargatze, R. F., Bishop, D. K., Orosz, C. G., Wu, N. W., and Butcher, E. C. (1989a). *Transplantation* **48**, 727–731.
Jutila, M. A., Lewinsohn, D. M., Berg, E. L., and Butcher, E. C. (1990). *In* "Leukocyte Adhesion Molecules" (T. A. Springer, D. C. Anderson, A. S. Rosenthal, and R. Rothlein, eds.), pp. 227–235. Springer-Verlag, New York.
Jutila, M. A., Rott, L., Berg, E. L., and Butcher, E. C. (1989b). *J. Immunol.* **143**, 3318–3324.

Kishimoto, T. K., Jutila, M. A., Berg, E. L., and Butcher, E. C. (1989). *Science* **245**, 1238–1241.

Kishimoto, T. K., Jutila, M. A., and Butcher, E. C. (1990). *Proc. Natl. Acad. Sci. U.S.A.* **87**, 2244–2248.

Kruschwitz, M., Fritzsche, G., Schwaring, R., Micklem, K., Mason, D. Y., Falini, B., and Stein, H. (1991). Submitted for publication.

Lasky, L. A., Singer, M. S., Yednock, T. A., Dowbenko, D., Fennie, C., Rodriguiez, H., Nguyen, T., Stachel, S., and Rosen, S. D. (1989). *Cell* **56**, 1045–1055.

Lewinsohn, D., Bargatze, R., and Butcher, E. C. (1987). *J. Immunol.* **138**, 4313–4321.

Lowe, J. B., Stoolman, L. M., Nair, R. P., Larsen, R. D., Berhendt, T., and Marks, R. M. (1990). *Cell* **63**, 475–484.

McDermott, M. R., and Bienenstock, J. (1979). *J. Immunol.* **122**, 1892–1898.

Marchesi, V. T., and Gowans, J. L. (1964). *Proc. R. Soc. Lond. [Biol.]* **159**, 283–290.

Munro, J. M., Pober, J. S., and Cotran, R. S. (1989). *Am. J. Pathol.* **135**, 121–133.

Nakache, M., Berg, E. L., Streeter, P. R., and Butcher, E. C. (1988). *Nature (London)* **337**, 179–181.

Ohmori, K., Yoneda, T., Ishihara, G., Shigeta, K., Hirashima, K., Kanai, M., Itai, S., Sasaoki, T., Arii, S., and Arita, H. (1989). *Blood* **74**, 255–261.

O'Neill, J. K., Butter, C., Baker, D., Gschmeissner, S. E., Kraal, G., Butcher, E. C., and Turk, J. L. (1991). *Immunology* **72**, 520–525.

Ord, D. C., Ernst, T. J., Zhou, L. J., Rambaldi, A., Spertini, O., Griffin, J., and Tedder, T. (1990). *J. Biol. Chem.* **265**, 7760–7767.

Phillips, M. L., Nudelman, E., Gaeta, F. C. A., Perez, M., Singhai, A. K., Hakomori, S.-I., and Paulson, J. C. (1990). *Science* **250**, 1130–1132.

Picker, L. J., de los Toyos, J., Telen, M. J., Haynes, B. F., and Butcher, E. C. (1989). *J. Immunol.* **142**, 2046–2051.

Picker, L. J., Kishimoto, T. K., Warnock, R. A., Smith, C. W., and Butcher, E. C. (1991). *Nature (London)* **349**, 796–799.

Picker, L. J., Michie, S. A., Rott, L. S., and Butcher, E. C. (1990a). *Am. J. Pathol.* **136**, 1053–1068.

Picker, L. J., Terstappen, L. W. M. M., Rott, L. S., Streeter, P. R., Stein, H., and Butcher, E. C. (1990b). *J. Immunol.* **145**, 3247–3255.

Pober, J. S., Bevilacqua, M. P., Mendrick, D. L., Lapierre, L. A., Fiers, W., and Gimbrone, M. A., Jr. (1986). *J. Immunol.* **136**, 1680–1687.

Rasmussen, R. A., Chin, Y.-H., Woodruff, J. J., and Easton, T. G. (1985). *J. Immunol.* **135**, 19–24.

Reichert, R. A., Gallatin, W. M., Butcher, E. C., and Weissman, I. L. (1983) *J. Exp. Med.* **157**, 813–827.

Rosen, S. D., Singer, M. S., Yednock, T. A., and Stoolman, L. M. (1985). *Science* **228**, 1005–1007.

Sackstein, R., Falanga, V., Streilein, J. W., and Chin, Y.-H. (1988). *J. Invest. Derm.* **91**, 423–428.

Sanders, M. E., Makgoba, M. W., Sharrow, S. O., Stephany, D., Springer, T. A., Young, H. A., and Shaw, S. (1988). *J. Immunol.* **140**, 1401–1407.

Schieferdecker, H. L., Ullrich, R., Weiss-Breckwoldt, A. N., Schwarting, R., Stein, H., Riechen, E.-O., and Zeitz, M. (1990). *J. Immunol.* **144**, 2541–2549.

Schmitz, M., Nunez, D., and Butcher, E. C. (1988). *Gastroenterology* **94**, 576–581.

Scollay, R. G., Butcher, E. C., and Weissman, I. L. (1980). *Eur. J. Immunol.* **10**, 210–218.

Siegelman, M. H., van de Rijn, M., Weissman, I. L. (1989). *Science* **243**, 1165–1172.

Stamper, H. B., Jr., and Woodruff, J. J. (1976). *J. Exp. Med.* **144**, 828–833.

Stevens, S. K., Weissman, I. L., and Butcher, E. C. (1982). *J. Immunol.* **128**, 844–851.

Stoolman, L. M. (1989). *Cell* **56**, 907–910.

Stoolman, L. M., Tenforde, T. S., and Rosen, S. D. (1984). *J. Cell. Biol.* **96**, 1535–1540.

Streeter, P. R., Berg, E. L., Rouse, B. T. N., and Butcher, E. C. (1988a). *Nature (London)* **331**, 41–46.

Streeter, P. R., Picker, L. J., Michie, S., and Butcher, E. C. (1991). *Cell Reg.* (in press).
Streeter, P. R., Rouse, B. T. N., and Butcher, E. C. (1988b). *J. Cell. Biol.* **107**, 1853–1862.
Streilein, J. W. (1983). *J. Invest. Dermatol.* **80 (Suppl.)**, 12s–16s.
Tedder, T. F., Isaacs, C. M., Ernst, T. J., Demetri, G. D., Adler, D., and Disteche, C. M. (1989). *J. Exp. Med.* **170**, 123–133.
Wayner, E. A., Garcia-Pardo, A., Humphries, M. J., McDonald, J. A., and Carter, W. G. (1989). *J. Cell. Biol.* **109**, 1321–1330.
Walz, G., Aruffo, A., Kolanus, W., Bevilacqua, M., and Seed, B. (1990). *Science* **250**, 1132–1135.
Yednock, T. A., Butcher, E. C., Stoolman, L. M., and Rosen, S. D. (1987). *J. Cell. Biol.* **104**, 725–731.

CHAPTER 7

Structure–Function Relationships of the CD44 Class of Glycoproteins

W. Michael Gallatin, Stephen J. Rosenman, Amir Ganji, and Thomas P. St. John

ICOS Corporation
Bothell, Washington 98021

I. Introduction

The major topic of this volume, regulation of traffic of mature leukocytes across vascular endothelium, is certainly a process to which CD44 contributes. The class of cell surface glycoproteins now collectively termed CD44 has been the subject of numerous independent lines of investigation spanning over a decade. Only a subset of these studies, however, has had leukocyte migration per se as its primary focus. In fact, this widely distributed set of molecules has been "discovered" many times by many investigators pursuing apparently unrelated topics, including thymocyte maturation, epithelial cell binding to the extracellular matrix, and lymphocyte activation to name but a few. Thus, a *variety* of names exist for the same set of molecules. Fortunately, during the last 2 years direct comparisons made possible by the isolation of genes encoding CD44 isoforms and through exchanges of antibodies between laboratories have reduced much of the confusion. Even so we expect that much of the earlier literature describing what turned out to be CD44-related phenomena will still be rather impenetrable to the non-CD44 student. While this chapter is not intended as a comprehensive review, it is our goal to make this field, both current and past, more accessible. Accordingly, an historical clarification of the nomenclature is provided first. The rest of our discussion is organized topically rather than chronologically. In particular, we have chosen to summarize the molecular genetic data on structure first because these influence interpretations of CD44's functional role in leukocyte traffic as well as other phenomena.

II. Historical Perspective and Previous Nomenclature

Typically the molecules described in early experiments are isoforms of CD44 in the 80 to 95 kDa range that are common to most cells. Although expression of CD44 epitopes on cells of nonhematopoietic origin was observed from the outset, CD44 was followed in many early studies primarily as a marker for leukocyte differentiation. Genetic data later revealed that epithelial restricted forms of CD44 with distinct core amino acid sequences existed (See next section).

Dalchau and co-workers first described the CD44 molecule in humans in 1980 using monoclonal antibody F10-44-2 and reported its differential expression on a subset of cortical thymocytes as well as a variety of other cell types. Hughes and August isolated a similar structure of 80 kDa from mouse fibroblasts cells in 1981. They coined the term phagocytic glycoprotein-1 (Pgp-1) because the glycoprotein identified was highly expressed on macrophages and granulocytes. Trowbridge *et al.* also discovered the same murine molecule, which they identified as a 95 kDa structure on granulocytes. They reported Pgp-1 expression on prothymocytes and granulocytic precursors as well as on lung, kidney, brain, liver, and cultured fibroblasts and described two allelic forms (Trowbridge *et al.*, 1982; Lesley and Trowbridge, 1982). Subsequently, the term Ly-24 has also been used to describe the murine antigen (reviewed in Holmes and Morse, 1988). That murine and human forms of CD44 would be highly homologous was also inferred prior to direct molecular genetic analyses: In 1986, Isacke *et al.* were able to identify a human homologue of Pgp-1 using a rat monoclonal antibody, IM7, that reacted with both murine and human cells. Haynes and colleagues (1983) identified an 80 kDa molecule, [In(Lu)] related p80, whose expression on erythrocytes was regulated by the autosomal dominant Lutheran blood group inhibitor gene (Telen *et al.*, 1983). Letarte *et al.* also found an identical structure on human B-cells (Letarte *et al.*, 1985). In fact, the identity between [In(Lu)] related p80, Pgp-1, F10-44-2 antigen, and the ECMRIII and Hermes receptors described later has been established in a number of laboratories (reviewed in Haynes *et al.*, 1990).

The first direct indication that CD44 might serve as an adhesion molecule for attachment to the extracellular matrix (ECM) was provided by Carter who identified a 90 kDa integral membrane glycoprotein on human fibroblasts (Carter, 1982) and subsequently demonstrated its affinity for types I and VI collagen and fibronectin (Carter and Wayner, 1988). This structure was termed extracellular matrix receptor type III (ECMRIII). Similarly, a plausible connection with leukocyte migration was provided by Jalkanen and her co-workers who reported that antibodies against the Hermes class of molecules interfered with the binding of human lymphocytes to mucosal high endothelial venules (HEV) *in vitro* (Jalkanen *et al.*, 1987). That these two phenomena, namely, binding of an ECM component and interaction of lymphocytes with HEV, were functionally connected was suggested by our finding that ECMRIII and Hermes were overlapping sets of molecules (Gallatin *et al.*, 1989; St. John *et al.*, 1990). This inference has been further strengthened by the identification of the primary structure of CD44 and by gene transfer experiments summarized in the next section.

III. General Structure of CD44

Although it is useful as a unifying nomenclature, the singular term CD44 is somewhat misleading because it refers to a collection of structural isoforms some of which are expressed preferentially on distinct cell types. Not all are derived simply by differential posttranslational modification of the same core peptide. While all share regions of high homology, at least two new versions incorporate unique elements of primary sequence, distinguishing them from their more "classical" relatives. It seems likely, therefore, that additional descriptors will be required in the future to specify each major isoform. With this in mind a brief description of the significant structural features of the known representatives of the CD44 class of adhesion molecules is provided here.

The major form of CD44 expressed by many cells of ectodermal and mesodermal origin consists of a 37 kDa polypeptide core that is covalently modified by addition of both N- and O-linked carbohydrate and sialic acid to yield a structure of 80 to 95 kDa Mr and by addition of chondroitin sulfate to give a larger 180 to 200 kDa form (Carter and Wayner, 1988; Jalkanen *et al.*, 1988; Omary *et al.*, 1988; Gallatin *et al.*, 1989; Stamenkovic *et al.*, 1989; Rosenman and Gallatin, unpublished data). Stamenkovic and co-workers' findings indicate that the lower molecular weight form also contains chondroitin sulfate (Stamenkovic *et al.*, 1991). Omary *et al.* also identified an intermediate species of 145 kDa that could have resulted from differential modification of the same core polypeptide or might have been derived from a distinct core sequence. Because their experiments predated molecular cloning of CD44, this question was not resolved. The relative proportions of these three forms vary among different cell types (Omary *et al.*, 1988), as does the degree of phosphorylation on serine residues (Isacke *et al.*, 1986; Carter and Wayner, 1988; Rosenman and Gallatin, in preparation). Finally, the tertiary structure of CD44 is modified by intrachain disulfide linkages formed among cysteines located in the N-terminal region (Goldstein *et al.*, 1989).

Molecular cloning of genes encoding CD44 has permitted additional inferences regarding the primary and secondary structure of this molecule and its probable functions. Early studies had already genetically mapped serologic expression of CD44 to chromosome 2 near the Ly-m11 gene in the mouse and the short arm of chromosome 11 in man (Lesley and Trowbridge, 1982; Francke *et al.*, 1983). The role of the In(Lu) gene in regulating expression of both the Lutheran antigen and CD44 on erythrocytes was also described (Telen *et al.*, 1983). Tentative assignments for the location within murine CD44 of allotypic epitopes have been made (Nottenburg *et al.*, 1989; St. John, unpublished data). In fact, prokaryotic and eukaryotic expression screening protocols as well as cross-hybridization schemes have been used to isolate CD44 cDNAs in man (Goldstein *et al.*, 1989; Stamenkovic *et al.*, 1989), baboon (Idzerda *et al.*, 1989), mouse (Nottenburg *et al.*, 1989; Zhou *et al.*, 1989; Wolffe *et al.*, 1990), rat (Gunthertt *et al.*, 1991), dog (B. Sandmaier, personal communication), hamster (Aruffo *et al.*, 1990), and bovine systems (Bosworth *et al.*, 1990).

The major structural features of all these versions of CD44 are similar with a high degree of amino acid sequence homology in evidence in both the internal and external domains (Fig. 1A). As a representative case, the human gene predicts a short hydrophobic leader followed by an extracellular domain of 248 amino acids, a 21 amino acid hydrophobic putative transmembrane region, and a 72 amino acid C-terminal cytoplasmic tail (Stamenkovic *et al.*, 1989). Goldstein and colleagues (1989) reported a cDNA that would encode a CD44 molecule with a truncated cytoplasmic domain. This cDNA species could be indicative of a novel protein with distinct functions or may represent an incompletely spliced mRNA. Probable locations of the aforementioned posttranslational modifications with the mature molecule are suggested from the primary sequence data. The seven potential N-linked glycosylation sites are located primarily towards the N-terminal region while O-linked glycosylation most likely takes place in the membrane proximal portion of the extracellular domain. Similarly, the four Ser-Gly motifs forming potential chondroitin sulfate addition sites are located in the more carboxyterminal region of the external domain. The relative positions of these sites for covalent modification are conserved between animal species. The cytoplasmic portion contains 7 serines and 2 threonines but no tyrosines as potential sites of phosphorylation. Only serine phosphorylation has been reported. The canine sequence does contain a tyrosine substitution at position 344 relative to the human sequence, but there is no evidence that this residue is phosphorylated. The precise roles each of these secondary structural modifications plays in modifying CD44 function are largely undetermined.

A major inference derived from the molecular clone data has been that CD44 bears homology at its N-terminus to cartilage link proteins (Stamenkovic *et al.*, 1989; Goldstein *et al.*, 1989). The latter bind proteoglycan core proteins in cartilage, native collagen, and hyaluronic acid, and foster the formation of large proteoglycan containing aggregates (Chandrasekhar *et al.*, 1983). This finding was consistent with Carter's earlier data implying a role for CD44 in adherence to the extracellular matrix and suggested potential ECM ligands.

Interestingly, while this N-terminal region and the cytoplasmic domain are highly conserved (80 to 90%) between various animal species, the region of the extracellular domain proximal to the putative transmembrane region is much more divergent with approximately 35% homology seen between murine and primate forms (Fig. 1A). Perhaps not surprisingly, two of the three immunodominant epitopes of CD44 seen on cells of hematopoietic origin map to this region (Goldstein *et al.*, 1989). Given that CD44 almost certainly performs similar tasks in every animal, one might assume *a priori* that the high degree of variability allowed in the membrane proximal region means that large, unique sequence motifs in this part of CD44 are not critical for adhesive or other functions. However, other results obtained in functional assays using antibodies as probes may contradict this notion (See following section).

IV. Novel CD44 Isoforms

Based on immunochemical and genetic data three groups proposed that cells of epithelial origin might express novel forms of CD44 containing a distinct core peptide sequence. Picker and co-workers identified a 140 to

A

```
         1       10        20            30        40        50
  HUMAN  MDKFWWHAAWGLCLVPLSLA....QIDLNITCRFAGVFHVEKNGRYSISRTEAADLCKAF
 BABOON        R        Q    ....          E IY
 CANINE     LG  L      LR    ....         Y
 BOVINE    T   R        Q    ....         Y               K
  MOUSE         T      LQ    HPHQ     V   Y                       Q
HAMSTER                L     H..E         Y                       Q

           60        70        80        90       100        110
  HUMAN  NSTLPTMAQMEKALSIGFETCRYGFIEGHVVIPRIHPNSICAANNTGVYIL.TYNTSQYD
 BABOON                                                     . S
 CANINE             R   V                   Q  A     H      .IS
 BOVINE             A RN                                    . S
  MOUSE         D KL    K            N         A     H      V S   H
HAMSTER         D VM    K                   Q  A     H      . S   H

           120       130       140       150       160       170
  HUMAN  TYCFNASAPPEEDCTSVTDLPNAFDGPITITIVNRDGTRYVQKGEYRTNPEDIYPS....
 BABOON            G                              K           N  ....
 CANINE                      H                     S            N  ....
 BOVINE   I        G             E               TK           N  VVSP
  MOUSE                        S    V            SK     HQ   DA  ....
HAMSTER           L            S E  V            SK     HQ   DA  ....

                180       190        200       210       220
  HUMAN  .NPTDDDVSSGSSSERSSTSGGYIFYT.FSTVHPIPDEDSPWITDSTDRIPATRDQDT.F
 BABOON  .S                 L      NH   SP      G         T      GA.
 CANINE  .                TSA YK  H HLP AY TE Q  SRVSSNS HT I K H SSV
 BOVINE  SS P  EM    P    TSG YS  H HLP    SRPRR.  .SQRAENTSD   YGSSH
  MOUSE  . II        TI K TPES.  LH YLP EQ TG Q DSFFIR ...TL    R SSK
HAMSTER  . T            K TSG . V H YLP I STA Q D YFIG ...TM      SSM

                   240       250       260       270       280
  HUMAN  HPSGGSHT.THESESDGHSHGSQEGGANTTSGPIRTPQIPEWLIILASLLALALILAVCI
 BABOON  D       .  G   A      R          L
 CANINE     ER   .  G   A   S             M K                  V
 BOVINE  D   R Y .  A   A   S  E H        M K
  MOUSE  DSR S R V  G  LA   SAN DS VT     M R
HAMSTER  D R N L V DG KLTE  S N DS L S  R GGK RV     V

         290       300       310       320       330       340
  HUMAN  AVNSRRRCGQKKKLVINSGNGAVEDRKPSGLNGEASKSQEMVHLVNKESSETPDQFMTAD
 BABOON                   N         S
 CANINE                   N     G      I                 P      YT
 BOVINE                   N   TM E                      G
  MOUSE                   G   T       E                  P      C
HAMSTER                       K       E                  P

         350       360
  HUMAN  ETRNLQNVDMKIGV
 BABOON
 CANINE
 BOVINE
  MOUSE        S
HAMSTER
```

B

RTNMDSSHST TLQPTANPNT GLVEDLDRTG PLSMTTQQSN SQSFSTSHEG LEEDKDHPTT 60

STLTSSNRND VTGGRRDPNH SEGSTHLLEG YTSHYPHTKE SRTFIPVTSA KTGSFGVTAV 120

TVGDSNSNVN RSLSG 135

C

IATTPWVSAH TKQNQERTQW NPIHSNPEVL LQTTTRMTDI DRNSTSAHGE NWTQEPQPPF 60

NNHEYQDEEE TPHATSTTWA DPNSTTEEAA TQKEKWFENE WQGKNPPTPS EDSHVTEGTT 120

ASAHNNHPSQ RMTTQSQEDV SWTDFFDPIS HPMGQGHQTE SK 162

FIGURE 1

(A) Alignment of predicted amino acid sequences for CD44 from different species. Alignments and gap priorities are set relative to the human sequence with only amino acid differences shown for other species. Gaps are indicated by dashes. The putative transmembrane region is boxed. (B) Sequence of the inserted domain of human epithelial CD44. (C) Sequence of the inserted domain expressed in highly metastatic rat carcinoma cells.

160 kDa form in squamous epithelial cells that unlike the 90 kDa form isolated from lymphoid and glial cells, failed to interact with purified mucosal addressin (Picker *et al.*, 1989; also reviewed in this volume). Similarly, Kansas *et al.* (1989) found that exhaustive glycosidase digestions of CD44 isolated from keratinocytes and lymphoid cells did not yield proteins of identical electrophoretic mobilities. Using a molecular genetic approach Stamenkovic and colleagues identified novel transcripts expressed weakly in epithelial cells and at high levels in some carcinomas (Stamenkovic *et al.*, 1989). We also found evidence for tissue selective expression of distinct CD44 related mRNAs (St. John *et al.*, 1989). Two groups reported human cDNAs corresponding to at least one of these transcripts that are expressed selectively in epithelial cells. The essentially identical genes isolated by both Brown and colleagues (1991) and Stamenkovic and associates (1991) are the same as those previously isolated for CD44 with the notable exception being the incorporation of additional 132 to 135 amino acid domains (Fig. 1B) beginning at positions 221 and 223, respectively, of the human sequence. The insertion falls within the minimally conserved, membrane proximal portion of the external domain. These are assumed to be the products of differential mRNA splicing with the minor differences between them (e.g., a two amino acid deletion at the

upstream insertion and a glutamic acid to glycine substitution at the downstream insertion) generated during the splicing process. The inserted sequence bears no homology to the other regions of CD44 or to other sequences in the data base. All the functional consequences of this insertion are not clearly delineated. It is clear, however, that the product of this gene is coexpressed on some epithelial cells along with the 90 kDa form found also in hematopoietic cells. Expression of this new gene in transfectants yielded a mature protein of approximately 130 kDa Mr. Further, Stamenkovic *et al.* (1991) have shown that cells transfected with the original "hematopoietic" CD44 cDNA (CD44H) bind hyaluronate better than do cells given the epithelial version (CD44E). Whether CD44E binds a different ligand or promotes an entirely different function (for example, association with another molecule in the plasma membrane) will undoubtedly be determined.

In addition to the two core peptide isoforms already described, another version of CD44 was described in a highly metastatic rat carcinoma (Gunthertt *et al.*, 1991). It also is distinguished by insertion at the same location (relative to the human sequence) of an additional domain consisting of 162 amino acids (Fig. 1C). In this case a reciprocal small deletion of the original sequence between positions 223 and 247 was found. Although the rest of the rat protein has the usual homology pattern with CD44s in other species, the inserted sequence bears no obvious sequence similarity to the rest of the rat CD44 molecule or, more importantly, to the aforementioned 135 amino acid insert seen in human epithelium. Given this information and the lack of positive functional data for CD44E, it is impossible to determine whether the rat and human inserts are functional homologues whose sequences have simply diverged or if the rat sequence represents yet a third CD44 isoform whose true counterpart in man has yet to be described. Related to this point, Gunthertt *et al.* (1991) used a probe specific to the rat inserted sequence to detect complementary mRNAs in normal lung, plastic-adherent blood leukocytes, and in peritoneal exudate cells. Although the exact cellular origin of the mRNAs was not determined, it seems likely that they might be derived from macrophages. This would be somewhat at variance with the apparent epithelial restriction of CD44E in man. Therefore, to avoid confusion, a degree of caution should be observed in the early classification of these CD44 isoforms. Multiple distinct CD44 related transcripts have been identified in cell lines and normal tissues (St. John *et al.*, 1989; Stamenkovic *et al.*, 1989; Gunthertt *et al.*, 1991). By analogy with NCAM, which undergoes developmental regulation through extensive mRNA processing (Santoni *et al.*, 1989), other as yet uncharacterized CD44 transcripts may encode novel proteins.

V. Direct Evidence of CD44 Adhesive Function

Substantial evidence has accumulated that CD44 acts both directly through ligand binding and indirectly through activation of other CAMs to promote adhesion both to the extracellular matrix and between homotypic and heterotypic cells. Its implication in leukocyte traffic phenomena came largely from Butcher and co-workers who reported that antiHermes antibodies blocked lymphocyte adhesion to specialized blood vessels, HEV, that normally support a high level of lymphocyte traffic (Jalkanen *et al.*, 1987). Consistent with their findings, we found that, among peripheral blood lymphocytes, the level of CD44 expression correlated with the capacity to bind cytokine activated endothelium *in vitro* (Fig. 2). In human lymphoid tissues the Hermes (CD44) antigens have a similar, though not identical, distribution to that observed for the prototype lymph node homing receptor, the MEL-14 antigen (Gallatin *et al.*, 1983). The two structures also share a similar molecular weight with a report of serologic cross-reactivity between them (Jalkanen *et al.*, 1987). Now that both have been molecularly cloned, it is obvious that they are completely unrelated structures. The true human homologue of MEL-14 is the Leu-8 antigen (also known as LAM-1 and LECAM-1), and both are members of the LECAM family of mammalian lectins (also reviewed in this volume).

In keeping with these observations we did not observe a significant increase in the ability of murine cells transfected with a primate lymphocyte CD44 to adhere to either HEV in any lymphoid tissue. However, we did observe that mouse fibroblasts (L-cells) transfected with this gene aggregated more readily than did the parent line when placed in suspension (St. John *et al.*, 1990). The aggregation was calcium independent and inhibitable by antibodies to primate CD44. Further, the capacity to aggregate depended on expression of the transfected genes because low expressing revertants selected from a transfected clone aggregated poorly. Homophilic binding between CD44 molecules on different cells was not an obligatory component of this adhesive behavior but involved CD44 recognition of a nonself-ligand because mixtures of parental and transfected cells formed heteroaggregates. We hypothesized that the ligand was an extracellular matrix component made constitutively by the parent line.

A number of groups have now demonstrated that one ligand of CD44 is, in fact, hyaluronate. Tarone *et al.* (1984) and Underhill *et al.* (1987) first reported an antibody, K-3, to an 85 kDa protein that inhibited hyaluronate (HA) binding to hamster kidney cells. Subsequently, this antigen was shown to be CD44 (Aruffo *et al.*, 1990). Similarly, Leslie and colleagues

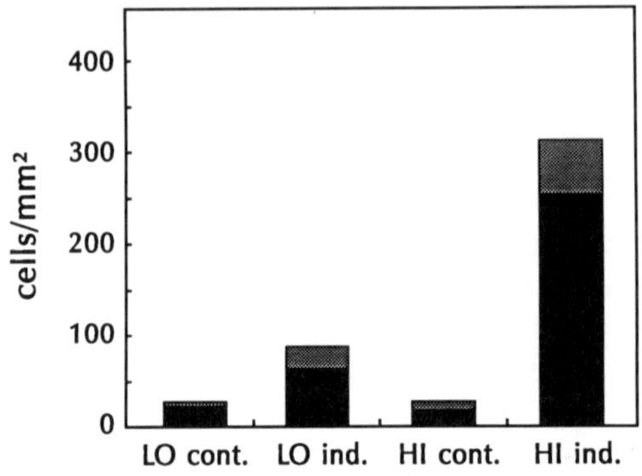

FIGURE 2

Correlation of CD44 expression on normal peripheral blood lymphocytes and *in vitro* adhesion to cytokine activated endothelium. Macaque lymphocytes were fractionated into CD44Lo (LO) and CD44Hi (HI) subsets by fluoresceinated cell sortings and incubated on monolayers of control (cont.) and IL4 induced (IND) macaque lymph node microvascular endothelium. ▦, Standard deviation; ■, mean.

(1990) described CD44 dependent binding of HA to mouse lymphoid cells. Moreover, Miyake suggested CD44 participation in HA dependent binding of lymphopoietic and myelopoietic precursors to bone marrow stroma (Miyake *et al.*, 1990a,b). We also found that addition of HA to primate CD44 transfected L-cells increased the size of aggregates formed (St. John and Gallatin, unpublished data).

The most direct evidence for binding of HA to CD44 was provided by Aruffo and co-workers who reported that soluble CD44 immunoglobulin chimeras bind to hyaluronate and to a lesser extent to other glycosaminoglycans. They found that immunohistologic staining of various tissues, including HEV, with this reagent was inhibited by hyaluronidase (Aruffo *et al.*, 1990). They also demonstrated differential binding of LECAM-1 negative lymphoblastoid cells transfected with the "hematopoietic" form of CD44 to rat lymph node stromal cells cultured *in vitro* (Stamenkovic *et al.*, 1991). The culture conditions used for the rat stroma were reported to maintain certain HEV characteristics *in vitro*. Regardless of the degree to which the cultured cells maintained organ specific "HEVness" in these experiments, the central point that CD44 fosters contact between heterotypic cells by binding HA was made. Also in this report, a polyclonal anti-CD44 antisera inhibited cell–cell binding, but the monoclonal antibody Hermes-3, previously reported to block adhesion to mucosal HEV (Jalkanen *et al.*, 1987), did not. This is interesting because the putative HA binding region of CD44 maps to the N-terminus while the Hermes-3 epitope localizes to the membrane proximal domain (Goldstein *et al.*, 1989). The implication of these data would be that the different regions of CD44 may bind distinct ligands.

VI. Effect of Cellular Context on CD44 Function

One paradox in our aggregation experiments was that mouse L-cells that make their own murine CD44 did not aggregate intrinsically. Because we assumed that primate and murine CD44s would have the same ligand specificity (not necessarily a valid assumption given the discovery of novel CD44 isoforms) we further hypothesized that the activity of CD44 vis-a-vis adhesion might depend on its interactions with other plasma membrane molecules or with intracellular components. If so, we reasoned that these associations might be species specific. To test this idea, chimeric molecules were made between the primate and murine CD44s consisting of reciprocally exchanged cytoplasmic and extracellular domains. In one set of experiments with transfectants expressing constructs, the ability to confer aggregation competence segregated with the primate cytoplasmic domain. However, subsequent transfection of these chimeric cDNAs into other cells including other clones of L-cells did not yield consistent results. These findings raise the possibilities that additional cellular components contribute to CD44 function and that these properties can segregate independently from CD44. Along these lines, Leslie *et al.* (1990) found that highly CD44 positive murine lymphoid cell lines were not always active in CD44 mediated hyaluronate binding. In some cases an activation step triggered by a phorbol ester was a prerequisite.

VII. Involvement of CD44 in Lymphocyte Activation

CD44 binding to its cognate ligand(s) may do more than simply promote lymphocyte adhesion directly. An additional function may be to provide the cell with information about its local environment (e.g., ECM contact) so that appropriate responses are made. If so, this could provide a mechanism whereby leukocytes in distinct anatomic compartments (for example, in the tissues versus in blood) could alter their thresholds for activation by other stimuli. This paradigm has been established for matrix adhesion mediated by the integrin, VLA-5 (Matsuyama *et al.*, 1989). In fact, we found CD44 levels on recirculating macaque lymphocytes varied as a function of anatomic compartment and were linked to cell cycle status as well as the capacity to become activated by mitogenic stimuli (Willerford *et al.*, 1989; 1990). Others have found that cross-linking of CD44 with antibodies can provide a costimulus with anti-CD2 and CD3 reagents for triggering T-cell proliferation and IL-2 synthesis (Shimizu *et al.*, 1989; Huet *et al.*, 1989; Denning *et al.*, 1990). In addition, a direct effect of anti-CD44 reagents to trigger IL-1 and TNF-alpha has been observed (Webb *et al.*, 1990; Denning *et al.*, 1990). Horgan and colleagues (1990) found that the degree of CD44-mediated augmentation varied with the paired costimulus (e.g., anti-CD3 versus a superantigen). Antibody mediated cross-linking of CD44 has also been shown to modify the function of other CAMS on the same cell. For example, LFA-1-dependent adhesion can be enhanced in this manner (Koopman *et al.*, 1990). Reciprocally, the amount and probably the adhesive properties of CD44 are increased as an early event during T-cell activation prior to S phase (Lynch *et al.*, 1987; Willerford *et al.*, 1989).

VIII. CD44 Expression on Memory T Cells

Although the specific signal transduction pathways involved in the events already described are not molecularly defined, we have found that in primates CD44 may be differentially phosphorylated on naive and memory T-cells (Rosenman *et al.*, in preparation). In both primates and rodents vigorous T-cell responses to recall antigens are linked with high level CD44 expression (Sanders *et al.*, 1988; Budd *et al.*, 1987). We found that in macaques the CD44hi, putative memory population expressed CD44 that was hypophosphorylated relative to naive cells. This condition and the relatively greater amount of CD44 on memory cells may or may not contribute directly to differential migratory properties of T-lymphocytes *in vivo*. Mackay and colleagues (1990) have found that T-cell subsets defined in this manner have distinct recirculatory pathways. The subpopulation containing memory cells trafficked selectively from blood into the tissues and accumulated in afferent lymph, while naive cells trafficked more frequently into efferent lymph, having entered the lymph nodes from blood via the HEV.

IX. Involvement of CD44 in Transmigration across Endothelium

In our earlier experiments we had found that CD44 transfectants did not bind appreciably better *in vitro* to HEV on tissue sections than did the parental cell lines. At face value, this result suggested that CD44 was not in and of itself sufficient to mediate HEV binding. Yet, as already mentioned, antibodies to the molecule can inhibit adhesion to endothelium (Jalkanen *et al.*, 1987; Oppenheimer-Marks *et al.*, 1990). One possible reconciliation of these facts would be a model wherein CD44 associates physically with another CAM, such as LECAM-1, that might play a more primary role in initial binding to endothelium. Thus, some anti-CD44 antibodies might be expected to block adhesion not by interfering with CD44 ligand binding per se but, rather, by perturbing activities of the associated structure.

To examine this possibility we asked whether or not CD44 associated selectively with other cell surface glycoproteins found on recirculating lymphocytes. In fact, in cocapping experiments wherein the location of each structure was visualized by laser scanning confocal microscopy we found evidence suggesting colocalization of CD44 with CD2, LECAM-1, and a subset of CD45R molecules (Rosenman *et al.*, in preparation). An example of this observation depicting CD44/CD2 association is shown in Fig. 3. The CD44/CD2 case is particularly interesting in light of the co-mitogenic activities mentioned earlier.

FIGURE 3

Co-capping of CD44 and CD2. Paired laser scanning confocal micrographs of normal macaque lymphocytes capped with biotinylated anti-CD44 plus Texas Red coupled avidin (right) subsequently stained with fluorescein conjugated anti-CD2 (left).

These types of associations were selective in that other integral membrane glycoproteins, such as CD4, did not show the same association. However, at this level of resolution it cannot be determined whether or not a direct molecular juxtaposition of CD44 and the other structures occurs. We have no biochemical evidence from coprecipitation experiments for direct contact between CD44 and these other molecules, although the report by Jalkanen *et al.* (1987) describing MEL-14/CD44 cross-reactivity may be evidence in this direction. Alternatively, it may be that the selective associations of transmembrane molecules we observed are mediated indirectly through similarly selective linkages involving specific cytoskeletal components. CD44 attachment to the cytoskeleton has been known for some time (Carter, 1982; Tarone *et al.*, 1984; Lacey and Underhill, 1987; Kalomiris and Bourguignon, 1988).

To examine the intramembrane topography of CD44 in a context more relevant to leukocyte traffic we asked whether or not this molecule was repositioned during transendothelial migration. Movement across an endothelial barrier is a complex process that can be viewed simplistically as a series of discrete steps in a temporal cascade (Fig. 4). *A priori*, CD44 could be involved in steps other than the initial binding to a lumenal surface. To test this we used a model system in which lymphocyte attachment to endothelium is mediated primarily by a VLA-4/VCAM-1 interaction (Masinovsky *et al.*, 1990). In this scenario, round lymphocytes, which have only recently become attached to endothelial cells, show a uniform CD44 distribution on their surface (Fig. 5A). Subsequently, the cells deform

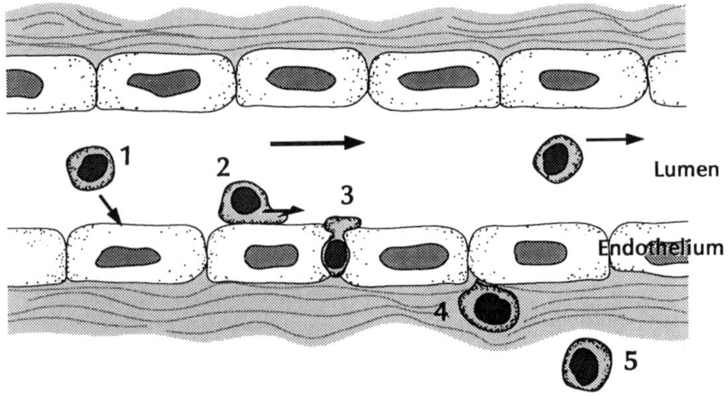

FIGURE 4

Schematic representation of steps in leukocyte transmigration across a small blood vessel. 1. attachment; 2. shape change and movement; 3. migration between endothelial junctions (migration directly through endothelial cells may also occur); 4. interaction with the basement membrane; 5. release.

dramatically, sending out projections along the endothelial surface. Concomitantly, CD44 and the cytoskeletal elements to which it is presumably connected reorganize, becoming focused in these projections (Fig. 5B; Rosenman *et al.*, in preparation). How causally related these events are to eventual transmigration is not firmly established, but we did observe that in cell lines that expressed VLA-4 (i.e., were competent to bind the endothelium), lateral movement on the endothelium was correlated with CD44 expression. Interestingly, in this system repositioning is selective because another CAM, LFA-1, did not reorganize in the same fashion but remained more globally distributed on the cell surface. Repositioning of CD44 and other CAMs was largely dependent on lymphocyte–endothelium contact and may depend on the specific nature of the initial lymphocyte adhesion. For example, the consequences of binding through VLA-4 may be different from binding by other mechanisms, such as that employing LFA-1. Oppenheimer-Marks *et al.* (1990), using a different endothelial culture activation protocol, implicated both CD44 and LFA-1 in the transmigration process.

X. CD44 Expression and Maturation of the Immune System

Besides its more obvious implications in traffic of mature leukocytes, the regulated expression of CD44 during hematopoiesis suggests a role in adhesive behavior of more primitive immune cell precursors. One of the earliest observations about CD44 was that prothymocytes in the bone marrow were enriched in CD44hi cells and that the most primitive cells in thymus were CD44hi (Trowbridge *et al.*, 1982; 1985; Isacke *et al.*, 1986). Later it became obvious that intrathymic expression of this antigen is biphasic, with both the most primitive and most mature thymocytes being CD44hi (Haynes *et al.*, 1983). Although there are differences in CD44hi frequency between primates and mice, this general pattern may be significant vis-a-vis cell traffic because these two populations represent cells that either have recently been mobile, arriving from the bone marrow, or are poised for movement into the periphery.

Expression of CD44 also correlates with maturational status among bone marrow precursors of other hematopoietic lineages. In both mice and humans the primitive myeloid progenitor cells are CD44hi while expression decreases on more committed granulocyte progenitors and is again up-regulated on mature granulocytes (Bauman and Chen, 1987; Kansas *et al.*, 1990; Lewinsohn *et al.*, 1990). Similarly, CD44 expression increases during the progression from committed B-cell progenitor to mature B-cell

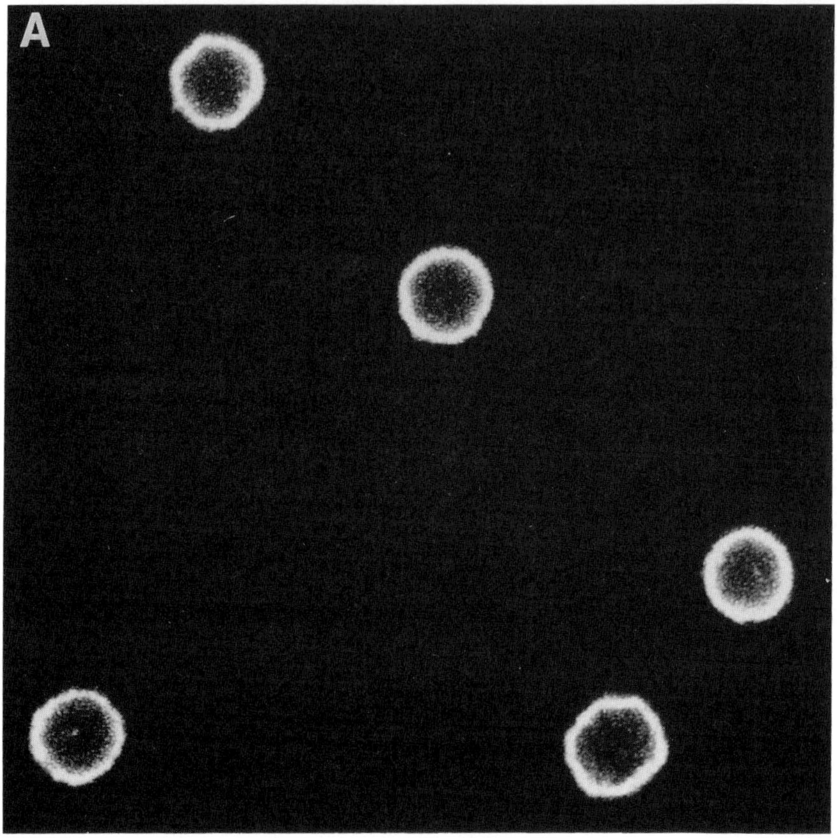

FIGURE 5

Topographical reorganization of CD44 during lymphocyte transmigration across endothelium. Confocal micrographs of CD44 distribution on lymphocytes (A) immediately before attachment to endothelium, and (B) after attachment to VCAM positive microvascular endothelium.

(Kansas *et al.*, 1990; Ryan *et al.*, 1990). That these observations may imply a functional role for CD44 during hematopoiesis is shown by the finding that anti-CD44 antibodies block B-lymphopoiesis *in vitro* (Miyake *et al.*, 1990a) and that hyaluronate blocks B-cell attachment to bone marrow stromal cells (Miyake *et al.*, 1990b). On a related theme, we found in a canine system that an antibody that facilitates *in vivo* survival of transplanted allogeneic bone marrow in irradiated recipients recognized CD44 (Schuening *et al.*, 1988; Sandmaier *et al.*, 1990). In this case, the mechanism of action is unclear. The antibody may effect homing of the infused graft, its interaction with the bone marrow microenvironment, or activity of a

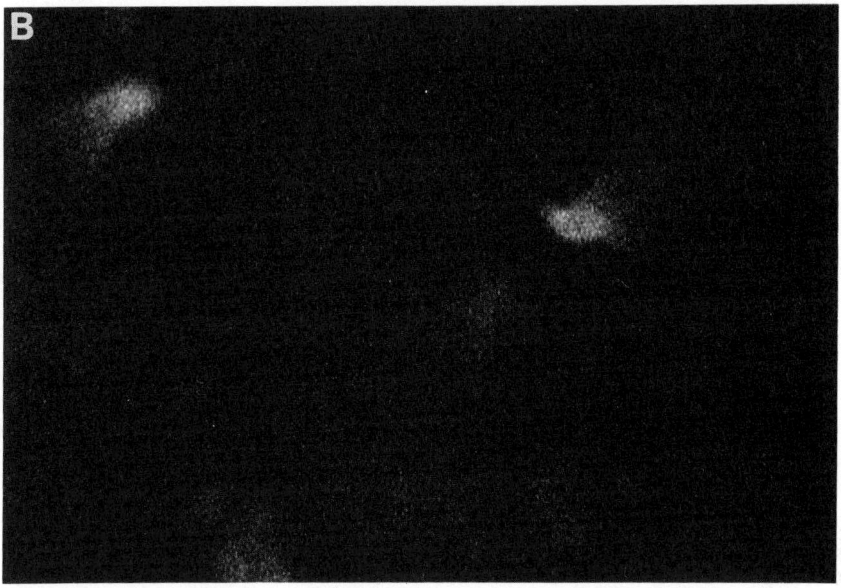

FIGURE 5 *(continued)*

radioresistant, CD44 positive host immunocyte (e.g., a natural killer cell) (Nagler *et al.*, 1989).

XI. CD44 and Metastasis

In addition to promoting the adhesive behavior of normal cells, CD44 may impinge on other pathologic processes. Many of the steps in extravasation of white blood cells during inflammation and in metastasis of neoplastic cells to secondary sites are conceptually similar and probably involve many of the same adhesive molecules. For example, the role of VCAM-1 and VLA-4 in adhesion to endothelium has been established for both normal lymphocytes and melanoma cells (reviewed in this volume). That CD44E is up-regulated in some transformed cells suggests its possible role in the metastatic process. This concept is further supported by the finding in a retrospective study of nonHodgkin's lymphoma that highly metastatic tumors typically bear higher levels of CD44 than do tumors that have failed to spread (Horst *et al.*, 1990). Unfortunately, probes to differentiate CD44 isoforms genetically were not available at the time these experiments were done. Nonetheless, Gunthertt and colleagues in an elegant series of experiments have obtained direct evidence for involvement of a specific CD44 isoform in metastasis (Gunthertt *et al.*, 1991). Using a rat model they selected highly metastatic variants of the carcinoma Bsp73ASML and raised a monoclonal antibody, MAb1.1ASML, that specifically recognized a metastatic variant but not the parental line. With this reagent as a probe they isolated from a prokaryotic expression library a cDNA encoding a portion of the antigen in question. Subsequent isolation of a full-length clone revealed that it encoded a version of CD44 containing the 162 base insert described earlier (Fig. 1C). Using a probe derived from the inserted region, they found that complimentary transcripts were only expressed in metastasizing carcinoma sublines. More significantly, transfection of the full-length cDNA into a nonmetastatic cell line converted it to the metastatic phenotype. Thus, a direct causal link between this isoform of CD44 and metastatic potential was established.

XII. Summary and Future Directions

CD44 is not a single molecular species, but, rather, it is a collection of molecules related, but distinct, in both primary structure and secondary modifications. Collectively, the class is involved in directing the movements and activation of primitive and mature leukocytes as well as metastasis of neoplastic cells. Through its recognition of hyaluronate and probably other ligands not yet defined it promotes linkage between the extracellular matrix and the internal cytoskeleton as well as adhesion among heterotypic cells. Some of these functions are accomplished indirectly through synergy with other cell surface glycoproteins.

Several very interesting questions remain to be answered about CD44. A few examples are:

1. Do CD44 molecules have more than on affinity state, and, if so, how are these states regulated?
2. Are there additional ligands with which CD44 interacts, and, if so, do they bind selectively to a particular CD44 isoform, CD44E, for example?
3. In molecular terms what signal transduction mechanisms trigger CD44 repositioning in the plasma membrane and its association with other cell surface glycoproteins?
4. Is CD44E the human counterpart of the molecule described by Gunthertt and co-workers (1991), and, if so, can inferences about its mode of action be used clinically to intervene in the metastatic process?

Hopefully, all of these will be resolved in the near future.

References

Aruffo, A., Stamenkovic, I., Melnick, M., Underhill, C. B., and Seed, B. (1990). *Cell* **61**, 1303–1313.

Bauman, J. G., and Chen, M. G. (1987). *Exp. Hematol.* **15**, 1074–1079.

Bosworth, B., St. John, T., Gallatin, M., and Harp, (1991). *Molecular Immunol.*, in press.

Brown, T. A., Bouchard, T., St. John, T., Wayner, E., and Carter, W. G. (1991). *J. Biol. Chem.* **113**, 207–221.

Budd, R. C., Cerottini, J. C., and MacDonald, H. R. (1987). *J. Immunol.* **138**, 1009–1013.

Carter, W. G. (1982). *J. Biol. Chem.* **257**, 3249–3257.

Carter, W., and Wayner, E. (1988). *J. Biol. Chem.* **263**, 4193–4201.

Chandrasekhar, S., Kleinman, H. K., and Hassell, J. R. (1983). *J. Biol. Chem.* **258**, 6226–6231.

Colombatti, A., Hughes, E. N., Taylor, B. A., and August, J. T. (1982). *Proc. Natl. Acad. Sci. U.S.A.* **79**, 1926–1929.

Dalchau, R., Kirkley, J., and Fabre, J. W. (1980). *Eur. J. Immunol.* **10**, 745–749.

Denning, S. M., Le, P. T., Singer, K. H., and Haynes, B. F. (1990). *J. Immunol.* **144**, 7–15.

Francke, U., Foellmer, B. E., and Hyanes, B. F. (1983). *Somatic Cell Genetics* **9**, 333–344.

Gallatin, W. M., Wayner, E., Hoffman, P., St. John, T., Butcher, E. C., and Carter, W. (1989). *Proc. Natl. Acad. Sci. U.S.A.* **56**, 4654–4658.

Gallatin, W. M., Weissman, I. L., and Butcher, E. C. (1983). *Nature (London)* **304**, 30–33.

Goldstein, L. A., Zhou, D. F., Picker, L. J., Minty, C. N., Bargatze, R. F., Ding, J. F., and Butcher, E. C. (1989). *Cell* **56**, 1063–1072.

Gunthertt, U., Hofmann, M., Rudy, W., Reber, S., Zoller, M., Haubmann, I., Matzku, S., Wenzel, A., Ponta, H., and Herrlich, P. (1991). *Cell* **65**, 13–24.

Haynes, B. F., Harden, E. A., Telen, M. J. (1983). *J. Immunol.* **131**, 1195–1200.

Haynes, B. F., Telen, M. J., Hale, L. P., and Denning, S. M. (1990). *Immunol. Today* **10**, 423–428.

Holmes, K. L., and Morse, H. C. (1988). *Immunol. Today* **9**, 334–350.

Horgan, K. J., Van Seventer, G. A., Shimizu, Y., and Shaw, S. (1990). *Eur. J. Immunol.* **20**, 1111–1118.

Horst, E., Meijer, C. J., Radaszkiewicz, T., Ossekoppele, G. J., Van Krieken, J. H., and Pals, S. T. (1990). *Leukemia* **4**, 595–599.

Huet, S., Groux, H., Caillou, B., Valentin, H., Prieur, A. M., and Bernard, A. (1989). *J. Immunol.***143**, 798–801.

Hughes, E. N. and August, J. R. (1981) *J. Biol. Chem.* **256,** 7023–7027.

Idzerda, R., Carter, W., Wayner, E., Nottenburg, C., Gallatin, M., and St. John, T. (1989). *Proc. Natl. Acad. Sci. U.S.A.* **56**, 4659–4663.

Isacke, C. M., Sauvage, C. A., and Hyman, R. (1986). *Immunogenet.* **23**, 326–332.

Jalkanen, S. T., Bargatze, R. F., de los Toyos, J., and Butcher, E. C. (1987). *J. Cell. Biol.* **105**, 983–990.

Jalkanen, S. T., Jalkanen, M., Bargatze, R., Tammi, M., and Butcher, E. C. (1988). *J. Immunol.* **141**, 1615–1623.

Kalomiris E., and Bourguignon, L.-Y. W. (1988). *J. Cell. Biol.* **106**, 319–327.

Kansas, G. S., and Dailey, M. O. (1989). *J. Immunol.* **142**, 3058–3062.

Kansas, G. S., Muirhead, M. J., and Dailey, M. O. (1990). *Blood* **76**, 2483–2492.

Kansas, G. S., Wood, G. S., and Dailey, M. O. (1989). *J. Immunol.* **142**, 3050–3057.

Koopman, G., van Kooyk, Y., de Graaff, M., Meyer, C. J. (1990). *J. Immunol.* **145**, 3589–3593.

Lacey, B. E. and Underhill, C. B. (1987). *J. Cell Biol.* **105,** 1395–1404.

Leslie, J., Schulte, R., and Hyman, R. (1990). *Exp. Cell Res.* **187**, 224–233.

Leslie, J., and Trowbridge, I. S. (1982). *Immunogenet.* **15**, 313–320.

Letarte, M. (1986). *Mol. Immunol.* **23**, 639–644.

Letarte, M., Iturbe, S., and Quackenbuch, E. J. (1985). *Mol. Immunol.* **22**, 113–119.

Lewinsohn, D. M., and Nagler, A., Ginzton, N., Greenberg, P., and Butcher, E. C. (1990). *Blood* **75**, 589–595.

Lynch, F., Chaudhri, G., Allan, J. E., Doherty, P. C., and Ceredig, R. (1987). *Eur. J. Immunol.* **17**, 137–140.

Mackay, C. R., Marston, W. L., and Dudler, L. (1990). *J. Exp. Med.* **171**, 801–817.

Masinovsky, B., Urdal, D., and Gallatin, W. M. (1990). *J. Immunol.* **145**, 2886–2895.

Matsuyama, T., Yamada, A., Kay, J., Yamada, K. M. *et al.* (1989). *J. Exp. Med.* **170**, 1133–1148.

Miyake, K., Medina, K. L., Hayashi, S., Ono, S., Hamaoka, T., and Kincade, P. W. (1990a). *J. Exp. Med.* **171**, 477–488.

Miyake, K., Underhill, C. B., Lesley, J., and Kincade, P. W. (1990b). *J. Exp. Med.* **172**, 69–75.

Nagler, A., Lanier, L. L., Cwirla, S., and Phillips, J. H. (1989). *J. Immunol.* **143**, 3183–3191.

Nottenburg, C., Rees, G., and St. John, T. (1989). *Proc. Natl. Acad. Sci. U.S.A.* **86**, 8521–8525.

Omary, M. B., Trowbridge, I. S., Letarte, M., Kagnoff, M. F., and Isacke, C. M. (1988). *Immunogenet.* **27**, 460–464.

Oppenheimer-Marks, N., Davis, L. S., and Lipsky, P. E. (1990). *J. Immunol.* **145**, 140–148.

Picker, L. J., Nakache, M., and Butcher, E. C. (1989). *J. Cell Biol.* **109**, 927–937.

Ryan, D. H., Nuccie, B. L., Abboud, C. N., and Liesveld, J. L. (1990). *J. Immunol.* **145**, 477–484.

Sanders, M. E., Makgoba, M. W., Sharrow, S. O., Stephany, D., Springer, T. A., Young, H. A., and Shaw, S. (1989). *J. Immunol.* **140**, 1401–1407.

Sandmaier, B. M., Storb, R., Appelbaum, F. R., and Gallatin, W. M. (1990). *Blood* **76**, 630–635.

Santoni, M. J., Barthels, D., Vopper, G., Boned, A., Goridis, C., and Wille, W. (1989). *EMBO J.* **8**, 385–392.

Schuening, F., Storb, R., Goehle, S., Meyer, J., Graham, T., Deeg, J., Appelbaum, F., Sale, G., Graff, L., Loughran, T. (1987) *Transplantation* **44**, 607-613

Shimizu, Y., Van Seventer, G. A., Siraganian, R., Wahl, L., and Shaw, S. (1989). *J. Immunol.* **143**, 2457–2463.

St. John, T., Gallatin, W. M., and Idzerda, R. L. (1989). *Reg. Immunol.* **2**, 300–310.

St. John, T., Meyer, J., Idzerda, R., and Gallatin, W. M. (1990). *Cell* **60**, 45–52.

Stamenkovic, I., Amiot, M., Pesando, J. M., and Seed, B. (1989). *Cell* **56**, 1057–1062.

Stamenkovic, I., Aruffo, A., Amiot, M., and Seed, B. (1991). *EMBO J.* **10**, 343–348.

Tarone, G., Ferracini, R., Galetto, G., and Comoglio, P. (1984). *J. Cell. Biol.* **99**, 512–519.

Telen, M. J., Eisenbarth, G. S., and Haynes, B. F. (1983). *J. Clin. Invest.* **71**, 1878–1886.

Trowbridge, I. S., Lesley, J., and Schulte, R. (1982). *Immunogenet.* **15**, 299–312.

Trowbridge, I. S., Lesley, J., Trotter, J., and Hyman, R. (1985). *Nature (London)* **315**, 666–669.

Underhill, C. B., Green, S. J., Comoglio, P. M., and Tarone, G. (19??). *J. Biol. Chem.* **B262**, 13142–13146.

Webb, D. S., Shimizu, Y., Van Seventer, G. A., Shawn, S., and Gerrard, T. L. (1990). *Science* **249**, 1295–1297.

Willerford, D. M., and Gallatin, W. M. (1990). *In* "Cellular Immunity and the Immunotherapy of Cancer" (M. Lotze and O. Finn, eds.), Wiley-Liss, New York.

Willerford, D. M., Hoffman, P. A., and Gallatin, W. M. (1989). *J. Immunol.* **142**, 3416–3422.

Wolffe, E. J., Gause, W. C., Pelfrey, C. M., Holland, S. M., Steinberg, A. D., and August, J. T. (1990). *J. Biol. Chem.* **265**, 341–347.

Zhou, D. F., Ding, J. F., Picker, L. J., Bargatze, R. F., Butcher, E. C., and Goeddel, D. V. (1989). *J. Immunol.* **15**, 3390–3395.

CHAPTER 8

Vascular Cell Adhesion Molecule-1

Roy Lobb, Catherine Hession, and Laurelee Osborn

BIOGEN, Inc.
Cambridge, Massachusetts 02142

I. Introduction

Leukocyte emigration through the vascular wall is a key characteristic of the inflammatory response, and an understanding of this process should provide new opportunities for therapeutic intervention (Harlan, 1985). Significant progress has been made in the molecular characterization of the initial part of this process, endothelial–leukocyte adhesion (Harlan, 1985; Stoolman, 1989; Osborn *et al.*, 1989; Osborn, 1990; Carlos and Harlan, 1990; Springer, 1990; Pober and Cotran, 1990; Brandley *et al.*, 1990). Three general mechanisms of adhesion have now been defined, rapid transient up-regulation of leukocyte adhesion molecules (e.g., CD11b/CD18)[1]; rapid

[1] Abbreviations: CD, cluster of differentiation; ELAM-1, endothelial leukocyte adhesion molecule-1; HUVEC, human umbilical vein endothelial cell; ICAM-1, intercellular adhesion molecule-1; VCAM-1, vascular cell adhesion molecule-1; GMP-140, granule membrane protein-140; VLA, very late antigen; PMN, polymorphonuclear leukocyte (neutrophil); LEC-CAM, lectin-epidermal growth factor-complement related cell adhesion molecule; IL, interleukin; TNF, tumor necrosis factor; Ig, immunoglobulin; CEA, carcinoembryonic antigen; NCAM; neural cell adhesion molecule; INCAM-110, induced cell adhesion molecule-110; CFD, carboxyfluorescein diacetate; Fn, fibronectin; LFA-1, lymphocyte function–associated antigen–1.

Cellular and Molecular Mechanisms of Inflammation, Volume 2

transient up-regulation of endothelial adhesion molecules (e.g., GMP-140); and more persistent cytokine activation of endothelial cells, leading to the synthesis of new adhesion molecules (e.g., ELAM-1). In addition, three families of adhesion molecules have emerged, the LECCAMs or SELECTINs (e.g., ELAM-1), which appear to interact with carbohydrate containing ligands; the heterodimeric integrins (for example, the CD11/CD18 family); and members of the immunoglobulin (Ig) superfamily. In this Chapter we discuss the Ig superfamily member vascular cell adhesion molecule-1 (VCAM-1), which is synthesized by endothelial cells after cytokine activation *in vitro*, is present on vascular endothelium at sites of inflammation *in vivo*, and interacts with the leukocyte integrin VLA-4. The VCAM-1/VLA-4 interaction may play a critical role in the recruitment of mononuclear leukocytes to inflammatory sites *in vivo*.

II. Characterization of a Novel Endothelial–Lymphocyte Adhesion Pathway

When we began our initial studies on endothelial–leukocyte adhesion, two cytokine induced endothelial cell adhesion molecules had been characterized and cloned, ICAM-1 and ELAM-1. ICAM-1 is found on many cell types, and its expression on vascular endothelium is strongly up-regulated by the proinflammatory cytokines IL-1 and TNF, both *in vitro* and *in vivo* (Pober *et al.*, 1986; Simmons *et al.*, 1988; Staunton *et al.*, 1988; Dustin and Springer, 1988; Cotran and Pober, 1988). ICAM-1 binds to a subset of the β2 integrins (Marlin and Springer, 1987) including LFA-1 (CD11a/CD18, found on lymphocytes and most other leukocytes), and Mac1 (CD11b/CD18, found on phagocytes). ELAM-1, initially defined by a monoclonal antibody that partially inhibited PMN adhesion to IL-1 treated HUVECs (Bevilacqua *et al.*, 1987), is a member of the LECCAM family of adhesion molecules, which are structurally related to mammalian lectins, epidermal growth factor, and complement regulatory proteins (Bevilacqua *et al.*, 1987; 1989; Brandley *et al.*, 1990; Osborn, 1990). ELAM-1 binds neutrophils, monocytes and related myelocytic cell lines but not most resting lymphocytes, unlike ICAM-1, which can bind all these cell types.

Data from a number of laboratories have shown that neither ICAM-1 nor ELAM-1 fully account for lymphocyte adhesion to cytokine treated HUVECs observed *in vitro*. Although the ICAM-1/LFA-1 pathway does play a role in lymphocyte adhesion, it has been well established that blocking mAbs to LFA-1 can only weakly inhibit the binding of lymphocytic cells to activated endothelium (Haskard *et al.*, 1986; Dustin and Springer, 1988). Furthermore, in patients genetically deficient in CD18, and hence expressing no leukocyte LFA-1, lymphocyte recruitment into inflammatory sites is essentially normal, despite profound defects in recruitment of phagocytic cells (Anderson and Springer, 1987), indicating the existence of an ICAM/CD18-independent adhesion mechanism for lymphocytes.

ELAM-1 was initially characterized as an adhesion molecule for phagocytes (PMNs and perhaps monocytes) but not for lymphocytes based on its failure to bind lymphocytic cell lines. It has been suggested to be most important in PMN recruitment during acute inflammatory episodes, based on the relatively transient induction kinetics of ELAM-1 *in vitro (Bevilacqua et al.*, 1987). However, subsequent studies have shown that mAbs to ELAM-1 partially inhibit purified T-lymphocyte adhesion to cytokine activated HUVECs (Graber *et al.*, 1990). We have also shown directly that both NK cells and a significant population of T-cells bind to ELAM-1 (Lobb *et al.*, 1991). Thus, ELAM-1 may well represent an LFA-1 independent pathway for mononuclear leukocyte recruitment *in vivo* under certain circumstances. Although lymphoblastoid cell lines such as Raji, Ramos, and Daudi do not bind to ELAM-1 expressed in COS cells (Bevilacqua and Gimbrone, 1989), these cell lines do bind avidly to stimulated endothelial cells by an ICAM/LFA-1 independent pathway. Using an expressible ELAM-1 cDNA cloned by direct expression (Hession *et al.*, 1990) and the anti-CD18 mAb 60.3 (Beatty *et al.*, 1983), we assessed the adhesion of various human leukemia cell lines to both HUVECs and ELAM-1 expressing COS cells, and evaluated their adhesion mechanisms. Some cell lines, such as JY (a B lymphoblastic line), bound to HUVECs only through CD18, consistent with previously published data (Dustin and Springer, 1988). Some, such as HL60 and U937 (myelo/monocytic lines) bound to HUVECs partly through ELAM-1 and partly through other pathway(s). Finally, most lymphocytic lines, such as Jurkat (T-cell) and Ramos (B-cell), bound through neither CD18 nor ELAM-1, proving clearly that another adhesion pathway was operative on cytokine treated HUVECs (Osborn *et al.*, 1989).

III. Direct Expression Cloning of VCAM-1

Having established the existence of a new adhesion pathway for lymphocytic cell lines, we set out to clone the endothelial cell adhesion molecule responsible by direct expression techniques. To obviate the need for antibodies to detect expressing clones we developed a new screening procedure based on cell–cell adhesion itself, which was used in conjunction with a subtraction technique to enrich our library for cDNAs of interest (Osborn *et al.*, 1989; Hession *et al.*, 1990). cDNA was prepared from HUVECs treated for 2.5 hours with maximal doses of IL-1 and cloned into the expression vector CDM8 (Seed and Aruffo, 1987). The library was screened with a radiolabeled cDNA probe generated by subtraction of IL-1 induced HUVEC cDNA against uninduced HUVEC mRNA, and a sublibrary of only IL-1 induced cDNAs was picked from this screen. The sublibrary was rescreened with probes for ELAM-1 and ICAM-1, leaving 125 clones that hybridized with the subtracted cDNA but not with ELAM-1 or ICAM-1. These clones were pooled in groups of five and each pool was transfected into COS cells by spheroplast fusion. Cells were then screened for adhesion to fluorescently labeled Jurkat or Ramos cells 48 hours following fusion (Fig. 1). Plates were screened visually by fluorescence microscopy and "rosettes" of cells adherent to a single COS cell were picked, plasmid rescued, amplified, retransfected into COS cells, and rescreened. One rosette from the initial screen yielded numerous large rosettes on the secondary screen. Six individual plasmids from this pool were analyzed by gel electrophoresis, and the largest, with a cDNA insert of 2.8 kb, was electroporated into COS cells. When panned with either Jurkat or Ramos cells, numerous large rosettes were found. This clone was designated clone 41, or VCAM-1/CDM8 (Osborn *et al.*, 1989).

The cDNA insert of VCAM-1/CDM8 is 2811 bp in length, and contains 106 bp of 5′ untranslated sequence, a 1941 bp open reading frame and 734 bp of 3′ untranslated sequence. Hydrophobicity analysis and comparisons with known cleavage patterns predicted a type I membrane protein with a 24 amino acid signal peptide, a 582 amino acid extracellular domain, a 22 amino acid transmembrane domain, and a short 19 amino acid cytoplasmic tail. The amino acid sequence of VCAM-1 was analyzed for homology to other proteins in the NBRF and NEW data bases using the FASTP program, and homologies were found to numerous proteins, all of the immunoglobulin superfamily. Members of this superfamily are characterized by the presence of one or more Ig homology regions, each consisting of a disulfide bridged loop that has a number of antiparallel β-pleated strands arranged in two sheets (Williams and Barclay, 1988; Hunkapillar and Hood, 1989). Three types of Ig homology regions (C, V, and H, also known as C1, V, and C2) have been defined, each with a typical length and consensus of amino acid residues at key positions relative to the two cysteines that form the disulfide link (Williams and Barclay, 1988; Hunkapillar and Hood, 1989). VCAM-1 was found to contain six Ig domains, all of the H type (Fig. 2). It can be placed within a subset of the Ig

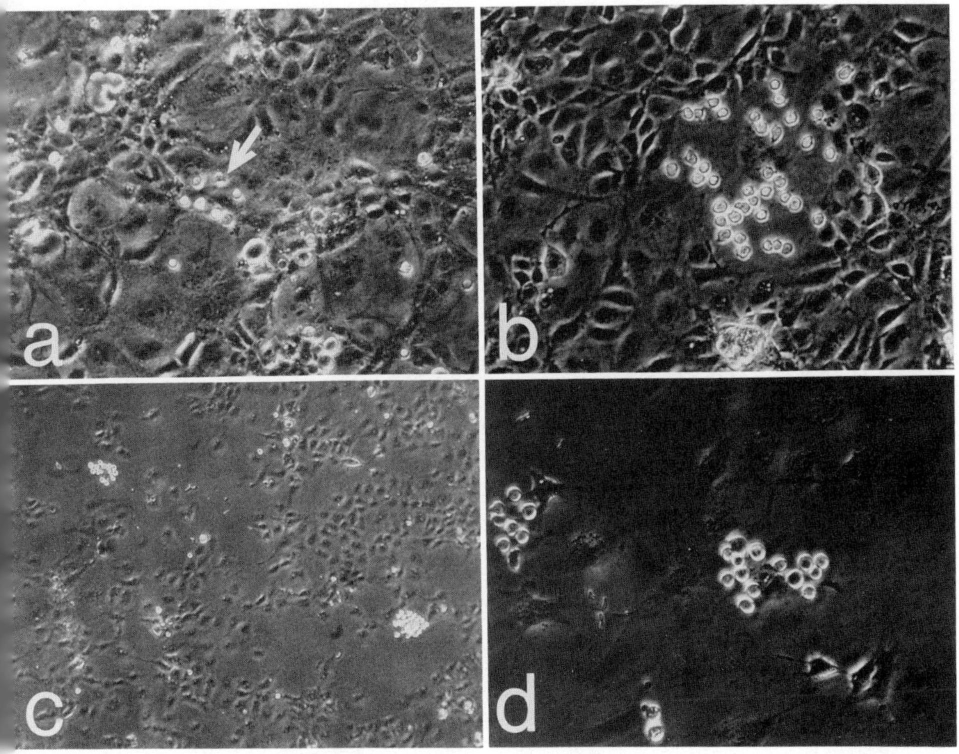

FIGURE 1

Functional detection and isolation of VCAM-1 cDNA clone 41. (a) COS cells transfected by spheroplast fusion with the induced HUVEC sublibrary were incubated with CFD labeled Ramos cells and washed (primary screen); the indicated small rosette was picked. (b) Plasmid DNA rescued from the rosette in (A) was electroporated into bacterial host cells and transfected by spheroplast fusion into COS cells, which were incubated with CFD labeled Ramos cells and washed as before (secondary screen); a representative of the resulting large rosettes is shown. (c) Plasmid minipreps were prepared from six bacterial colonies obtained from electroporation of the DNA rescued from the rosette in (A). The plasmid with the largest insert size (2.8 kb), clone 41, was electroporated into COS cells, which were panned as before. Numerous large rosettes were seen. (d) VCAM-1/CDM8 clone 41 electroporated into COS cells and panned with CFD labeled Jurkat cells. Each bar represents 100 μm. (Reproduced with permission from Osborn *et al.*, 1989.)

```
Clone #:
                                  *                                                  *
41  1E11               G  h f C       P  hWp                                p L f      DsG  o C   N
1    1          FKIETTPESRYLAQIGDSVSLTCSTTGCESPFFSWRTQIDSPLNGK-----------VTNEGTTSTLTMNPVSFGNEHSYLCTATCESRKLEKGIQVEIYS
2    2            FPKDPEIHLSGPL-EAGKPITVKCSVA-DVYPFDRLEIDLLKGDHLMKSQEFLEDADRKSLETKSLEVTFTPVIEDIGKVLVCRAKLHIDEMDSVPTVRQAVKEL
3    3      QVYISPKNTVISVNPSTKL-QEGGSVTMTCSSEGLPAPEIFWSKKLDNGNLQH------------LSGNATLTL-IAMRMEDSG-IYVCEGVNLIGKNRKEVELIVQ
     4         EKPFTVEISPGPRIAAQIGDSVMLTCSVMGCESPSFSWRTQIDSPLSGK-----------VRSEGINSTLTLSPVSFENEHSYLCTVTCGHKKLEKGIQVELYS
4    5       (A)FPRDPEIEMSGGL-VNGSSVTVSCKVP-SVYPLDRLEIELLKGETILENIEFLEDTDMKSLENKSLEMTFIPTIEDTGKALVCQAKLHIDDMEFEPKQRQSTQTL
5    6      YVNVAPRDTTVLVSPSSIL-EEGSSVNMTCLSQGFPAPKILWSRQLPNGELQP------------LSENATLTL-ISTKMEDSG-VYLCEGINQAGRSRKEVELIIQ
6    7        VTPKDIKLTAFPSESV-KEGDTVIISCTCGNV--PET-WIILKKKAETGDTVL-----------SIDGAYTIRKAQLKDAG-VYECESKNKVGSQLRSLTLDVQGREN

            NKDYFSPELLVLYFASSLIIPAIGMIIYFARKANMKGSYSLVEAQKSKV*
                       tm

                                                              f - aliphatic - L,I,V
                                                              h - hydrophobic - L,I,V,M,Y,F
                                                              o - aromatic - Y,F,W
                                                              p - polar - K,R,H,D,E,Q,N,T,S
                                                              s - small - A,G,S,T,V,N,D
```

FIGURE 2

Domain structure of VCAM-1. Domains present in clone 41 (six domain form) and clone 1E11 (seven domain form) are indicated. Conserved residues of Ig homology units of the H or C2 type are indicated at the top of the figure and underlined in each domain. (Adapted from Hunkapillar and Hood, 1989; Osborn *et al.*, 1989; and Hession *et al.*, 1991.) The alanine residue in parentheses (A) is not present in clone 1E11. The transmembrane region (tm) is underlined. Note the extensive homologies of domains 1 with 4, 2 with 5, and 3 with 6.

superfamily that contains other known adhesion molecules, including CEA, NCAM, and ICAM-1 (Hemperly *et al.*, 1986; Oikawa *et al.*, 1987; Simmons *et al.*, 1988; Staunton *et al.*, 1988; Williams and Barclay, 1988; Hunkapillar and Hood, 1989).

IV. An Alternate Form of VCAM-1

The VCAM-1 cDNA we originally isolated directs the expression of a functional adhesion molecule and encodes a protein containing six Ig homology units (Osborn *et al.*, 1989). Since then we have isolated a longer form of VCAM-1 (Hession *et al.*, 1991). The IL-1 stimulated HUVEC library previously generated (Osborn *et al.*, 1989; Hession *et al.*, 1990) was screened with radiolabeled VCAM-1 probe from our original clone encoding the six domain form of VCAM-1 and designated clone 41. Of three new clones isolated, two differed from clone 41 as assessed by restriction digests. One of these clones, 1E11, was sequenced and found to be identical to clone 41 except for an additional 276 nucleotides inserted between domains three and four of the original clone. This insert is predicted to encode an additional Ig homologous domain, which we have designated domain 4, renumbering the following domains 5 through 7 (Fig. 2). Domain 4 shows most sequence homology to domain 1. As we previously noted, domains 2 and 5, and 3 and 6, also show structural similarity. This implies that the basic unit represented by domains 1, 2, and 3 may have been duplicated at some point during evolution to give rise to 4, 5, and 6.

The insert is preceded by the nucleotides AAG, common to splice junctions. Thus, the two forms likely represent alternately spliced products of the same precursor RNA rather than the products of two different genes. This could occur most easily if the splice acceptor site of domain 4 is not optimal, resulting in skipping of this acceptor site in favor of the splice acceptor site of domain 5.

To discriminate between the two forms of VCAM-1 mRNA, we used the polymerase chain reaction (PCR) to amplify DNA fragments of different sizes representing the long and short forms. In an examination of HUVECs isolated from umbilical cords of individual donors, we found that both the long and short forms were induced in each of the three individuals tested and that the longer form predominates. As other laboratories have begun to clone VCAM-1 from the published sequence, both the longer seven domain form (Polte *et al.*, 1990) and the shorter six domain form (V. Dixit, personal communication) have been isolated, consistent with our data.

In summary, two alternative forms of VCAM-1 are induced by cytokine treatment of HUVECs *in vitro*. The structures of the cDNAs for these two forms suggest that they are products of the same gene and that the six domain form may be produced by the occasional skipping of the exon encoding domain 4 during splicing. Both forms support adhesion of VLA-4 expressing cells when expressed in COS7 cells (Hession *et al.*, 1991), indicating that domain 4 is not necessary for the adhesive function of VCAM-1. Whether or not this domain is important in other as yet undefined aspects of VCAM-1 function remains to be determined.

V. VCAM-1 Binds the Integrin VLA-4

In preliminary experiments to investigate the nature of the leukocyte ligand for VCAM-1, we found that the VCAM-1 dependent adhesion of Jurkat and Ramos cells was both temperature sensitive and energy dependent, consistent with the interaction of VCAM-1 with an integrin. Members of the integrin superfamily have been divided into three major subgroups (Hynes, 1987; Marcantonio and Hynes, 1988; Springer, 1990). The β2 integrins (LFA-1, Mac1, and gp150,95) are mostly involved in cell–cell interactions within the immune system (Kishimoto *et al.*, 1989), whereas members of the β1 and β3 integrin subfamilies predominantly mediate cell–matrix interactions (Hynes, 1987; Ruoslahti, 1988). ICAM-1, another member of the Ig superfamily, interacts with β2 integrins. As described previously, we had already eliminated β2 integrins as putative VCAM-1 ligands, because VCAM-1 dependent adhesion is not inhibitable by anti-CD18 mAb 60.3. The β1 integrin family, also termed the VLA proteins, includes at least six receptors that interact with the extracellular matrix proteins fibronectin, collagen, and laminin (Hemler, 1990). Unlike the other β1 integrins, VLA-4 is restricted to lymphoid and myeloid cells (Hemler, 1990), which are VCAM-1 binding cells. VLA-4 is known to be a receptor for fibronectin and has also been implicated in cell–cell interactions between lymphocytes (Hemler, 1990).

In collaborative studies with Martin Hemler and co-workers, we investigated the possible interaction of VLA-4 with VCAM-1 (Elices *et al.*, 1990). An anti-β1 antibody that blocks function of all the β1 integrins, as well as the specific anti-VLA-4 mAb HP2/1, completely blocked the adhesion of Ramos cells to either VCAM-1 expressing COS cells or to TNF stimulated HUVECs, implying that VLA-4 is indeed responsible for binding of Ramos cells to VCAM-1 (Fig. 3A,B). To confirm this indirect evidence, we examined VLA expressing stable cell lines for binding to VCAM-1. K562 erythroleukemic cells were chosen as host cells because they do not express surface VLA-4 and do not bind to either control or cytokine treated HUVECs. K562 cells do express VLA-5, however, allowing the expression of other VLAs by transfection with individual α chains, which can associate with endogenous β1. Thus, stable cell lines expressing either VLA-4 or, as a control, VLA-2, were generated. We found that VLA-4 expressing transfectants, but not control VLA-2 expressing transfectants or the K562 cells themselves, bound to VCAM-1 expressing COS cells, confirming directly the VCAM-1/VLA-4 interaction (Fig. 3C,D). Similar conclusions were reached independently using an established human CD11/CD18 deficient lymphoblastoid cell line and blocking mAbs (Schwartz *et al.*, 1990).

These and subsequent results suggest that VLA-4 is the major, and perhaps the only, receptor for VCAM-1. Cell types known to bind to VCAM-1, including HL60, Ramos, Jurkat, THP1, U937, Molt4, HPB-ALL, Raji, SK-Mel-24, human T-cells, monocytes, and T-blasts, all express VLA-4, while those cells that do not bind to VCAM-1, such as JY cells, human PMN, and K562 cells, do not express VLA-4 (Osborn *et al.*, 1989; Rice and Bevilacqua, 1989; Elices *et al.*, 1990; Rice *et al.*, 1990; Carlos *et al.*, 1991a; unpublished observations). Thus, we have found an absolute correlation between VLA-4 expression and ability to adhere to VCAM-1.

VLA-4 also mediates cell attachment to the CS1 site within the heparin II binding fragment of human plasma fibronectin (Wayner *et al.*, 1989). The VLA-4 expressing K562 transfectants described earlier and Ramos cells bind to a fibronectin fragment (Fn40) containing the CS1 site in a VLA-4 dependent manner (Elices *et al.*, 1990), and this interaction is completely inhibitable by soluble Fn40 (Fig. 4A). In contrast, the interaction of VLA-4 expressing transfectants or Ramos cells with VCAM-1 cannot be inhibited by soluble Fn40 (Fig. 4B,C). These results demonstrate that the VLA-4/VCAM-1 and VLA-4/Fn interactions are functionally distinct. It is possible that VLA-4 expressing mononuclear leukocytes may independently regulate these two adhesive functions during the inflammatory response *in vivo*. Thus, they may bind sequentially to VCAM-1 expressed on vascular endothelium and to fibronectin deposited at inflammatory sites.

VI. Monoclonal Antibodies to VCAM-1

Several laboratories have produced monoclonal antibodies (mAbs) to cytokine activated endothelial cells in order to study various normal or pathological processes. A number of these mAbs to previously unidentified endothelial cell antigens are now known to recognize VCAM-1,

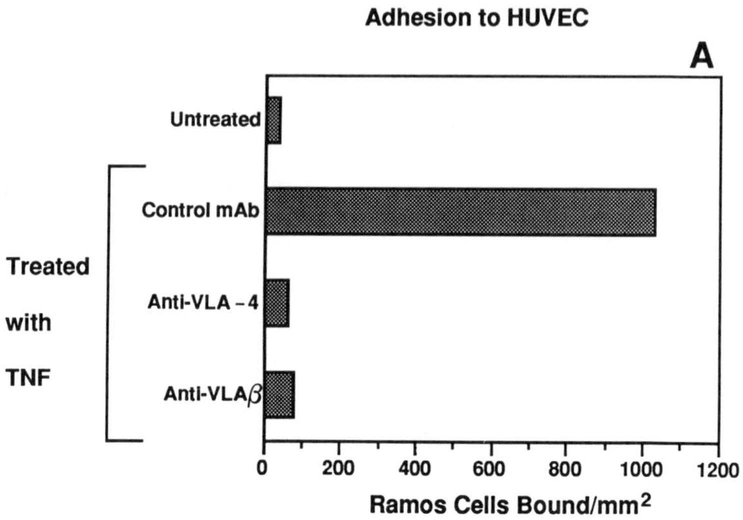

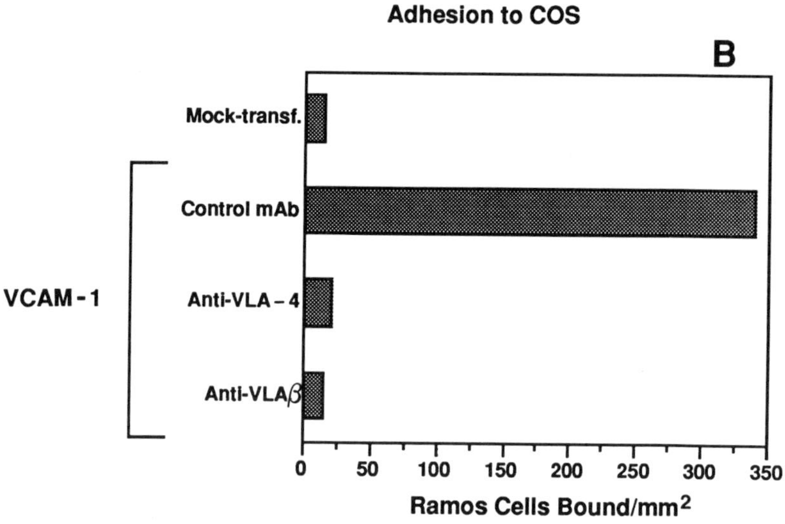

FIGURE 3

VCAM-1 binds the integrin VLA-4. Target cells (Ramos or K562 transfectants) were radiolabeled, and their binding to monolayers of HUVECs or transfected COS cells was assayed as described by Elices *et al.*, (1990). (A) HUVECs in 48 well plates were untreated or treated with 10 ng/ml TNF for 24 hours prior to assay. For inhibition experiments, target cells (Ramos) were preincubated for 20 to 30 minutes at room temperature with 5 to 20 μg/ml of mAb P3 (control), HP2/1 (anti-VLA-4), or B1E11 (anti-VLAβ1). (B) COS cells were electroporated with VCAM-1/CDM8 clone 41 and plated in 48 well plates 48 to 72 hours prior to assay, as described by

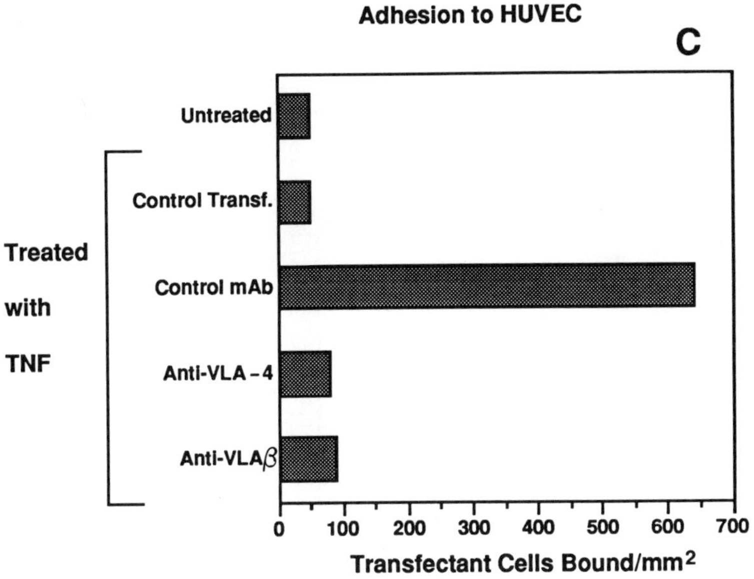

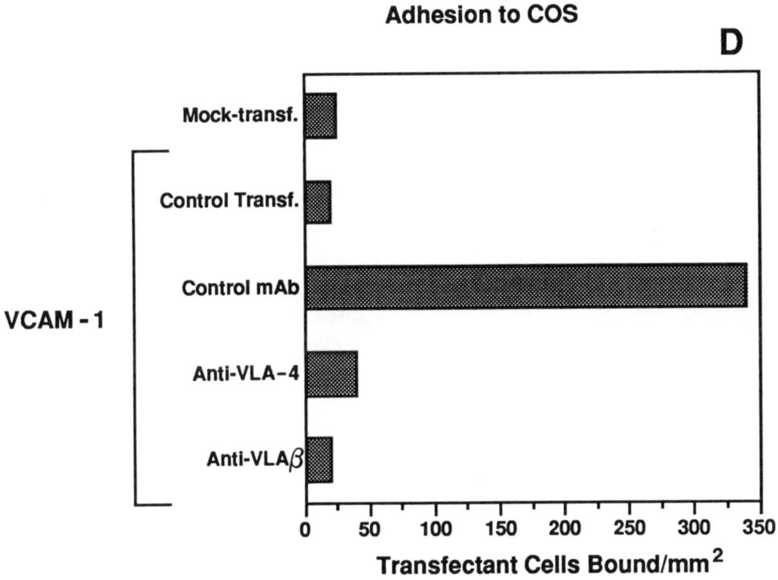

FIGURE 3 (continued)

Osborn *et al.*, (1989). Inhibition experiments were performed as in (A). (C and D) Stable K562 transfectants of VLA-2 (control transfectants) or VLA-4 (all others) were used as target cells in binding to untreated or TNF treated HUVECs (C) or mock versus VCAM-1 transfected COS cells (D). Inhibition experiments were performed as in (A). (Adapted from Elices *et al.*, 1990.)

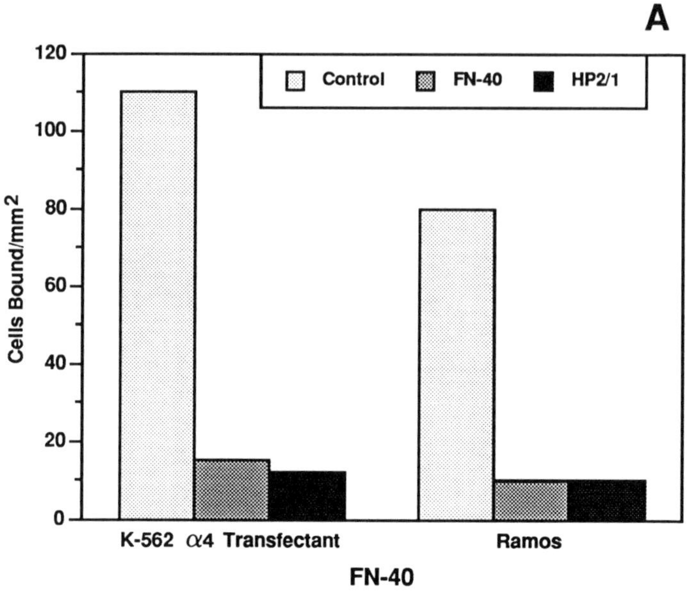

FIGURE 4

VLA-4 interacts with fibronectin and VCAM-1 by independent mechanisms. Adhesion of either K562 α4 transfectants or Ramos cells to (A) FN-40 (5 μg per well), (B) COS cells transfected with VCAM-1 clone 41, and (C) TNF activated HUVECs was carried out in the presence of soluble inhibitors: control (no addition); FN-40 (100 μg/ml); and mAb HP2/1 (anti-VLA-4). The binding assay was performed in serum-free medium. (Adapted from Elices *et al.*, 1990.)

including mAbs E1/6, 4B9, 1E7, 2G7, and 1.4C3, (Rice and Bevilacqua, 1989; Graber *et al.*, 1990; Rice *et al.*, 1990; Carlos *et al.*, 1990; Wellicome *et al.*, 1990).

Cytokine activation of endothelial cells *in vitro* increases the adhesion of human carcinoma and melanoma cell lines (Rice *et al.*, 1988; Dejana *et al.*, 1988; Rice and Bevilacqua, 1989). Although adhesion of the human colon carcinoma cell line HT29 to cytokine treated HUVECs (first shown by Dejana *et al.*, 1988) is mediated by ELAM-1 (Rice and Bevilacqua, 1989; Benjamin *et al.*, 1990), Rice and Bevilacqua showed that increased human melanoma cell adhesion to cytokine treated HUVECs was not caused by ELAM-1 or ICAM-1 (Rice and Bevilacqua, 1989). To identify endothelial surface structures involved in melanoma cell adhesion, mAbs were generated to TNF stimulated HUVECs. The mAb E1/6 recognized a novel,

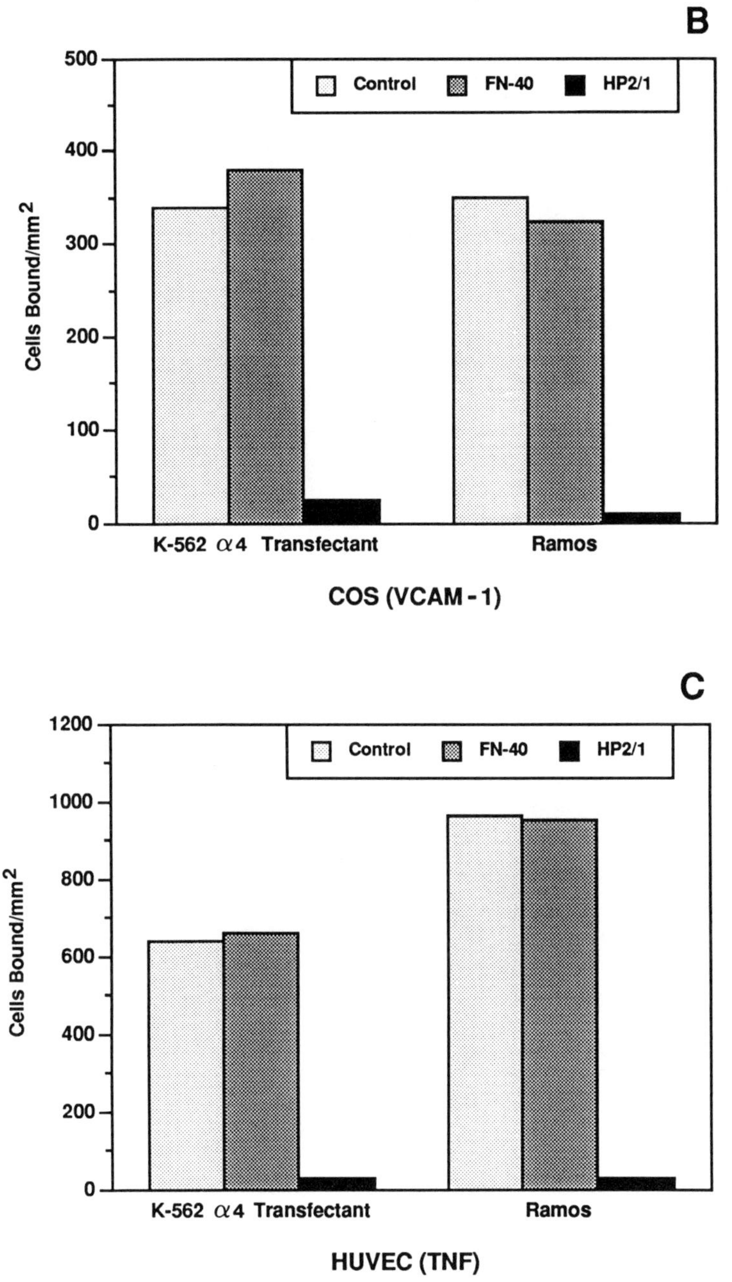

FIGURE 4. continued

inducible cell surface antigen that was shown to be responsible for melanoma cell adhesion and that was designated INCAM-110. Subsequent studies showed that INCAM-110 also supports monocyte and lymphocyte adhesion and that E1/6 recognizes an epitope encoded by the cDNA for VCAM-1 (Rice *et al.*, 1990).

mAb 4B9 was generated by immunizing BALB/c mice with HUVECs nonenzymatically harvested after treatment with TNF for 24 hours (Carlos *et al.*, 1990). Supernatants were screened initially by ELISA for selective binding to cytokine activated HUVECs and subsequently examined for inhibition of adhesion of KG1a cells, which bind to cytokine activated HUVECs by a largely LFA-1 independent pathway. mAb 4B9 inhibits the binding of Ramos, Molt4, KG1a, and PBL to TNF treated HUVECs. Its specificity for VCAM-1 was established by an ELISA screen of untransfected CHO cells and CHO cells stably transfected with ELAM-1, VCAM-1, or ICAM-1. mAb 4B9 reacted only with VCAM-1 transfected CHO cells.

mAbs 1E7 and 2G7 were generated from BALB/c mice immunized with 4 hour IL-1-stimulated HUVECs, and were two of a panel of mAbs selectively binding to IL1 activated HUVECs (Graber *et al.*, 1990). They were shown to bind to a novel inducible antigen distinct from ELAM-1 or ICAM-1, and mAb 2G7 was found to partially block the binding of highly purified T cells to activated HUVECs. Subsequently both 1E7 and 2G7 were shown to bind to VCAM-1 expressed in COS cells (Graber *et al.*, 1990).

mAb 1.4C3 was generated from mice immunized with 6 hour TNF-treated HUVECs and was one of a panel of mAbs that selectively bind to TNF-treated HUVECs (Wellicome *et al.*, 1990). mAb 1.4C3 does not affect lymphocyte adhesion to cytokine treated HUVECs but has been shown to recognize VCAM-1 (Thornhill *et al.*, 1991).

Studies with these mAbs and cytokine stimulated endothelium *in vitro* confirmed our results from northern analyses of VCAM-1 mRNA expression in TNF treated HUVECs (Osborn *et al.*, 1989). Cell surface VCAM-1 is detectable within 2 hours of cytokine stimulation, is maximal at 10 to 24 hours, and its expression is maintained for at least 72 hours in the continued presence of cytokine (Graber *et al.*, 1990; Rice *et al.*, 1990; Carlos *et al.*, 1990; Wellicome *et al.*, 1990).

VII. Expression of VCAM-1 *In Vivo*

Using the mAbs described in the previous section, a number of immunohistochemical studies have been performed to evaluate the pathophysiologic tissue distribution of VCAM-1 (Rice and Bevilacqua, 1989; Graber *et al.*, 1990; Rice *et al.*, 1990; Freedman *et al.*, 1990; Koch *et al.*, 1991; Carlos *et al.*, 1991b; Briscoe *et al.*, 1991). In general, little or no vascular staining of VCAM-1 has been found in normal tissues, although mAb E1/6 has been reported to stain a proportion of small blood vessels in normal lung, and focal expression has been reported in human tonsil and peripheral lymph node (Rice and Bevilacqua, 1989; Rice *et al.*, 1990). mAb 4B9 has been found to be consistently negative in all normal tissues examined, including lung tissue (J. Harlan, personal communication). In contrast, VCAM-1 is often expressed in inflammatory situations. E1/6 stains human vascular tissue in inflamed appendix, delayed hypersensitivity reaction, and insect bite (Rice and Bevilacqua, 1989; Rice *et al.*, 1990). 4B9 stains focally rheumatoid arthritic synovium (Koch *et al.*, 1991).

Later studies also show that VCAM-1 is expressed on the vascular tissue of rejecting human cardiac allografts, as assessed in endomyocardial biopsy tissues (Carlos *et al.*, 1991b; Briscoe *et al.*, 1991). mAb E1/6 stains arterial as well as venular endothelium, marking VCAM-1 as distinct from ELAM-1, which is expressed exclusively in venular endothelium (Cotran and Pober, 1988; Rice and Bevilacqua, 1989).

One of the most intriguing results obtained from these studies is that anti-VCAM-1 mAbs stain dendritic and macrophage-like cells in numerous normal tissues, including skin, synovium, and lymph nodes (Rice *et al.*, 1990; Freedman *et al.*, 1990; Koch *et al.*, 1991; Briscoe *et al.*, 1991; Griffiths *et al.*, 1991). In one report, functional assays were also performed, demonstrating the binding of VLA4-expressing activated human B-cells to INCAM110-expressing human follicular dendritic cells (Freedman *et al.*, 1990). The results suggest that the VCAM-1/VLA-4 pathway may play an important role in some aspects of the immune response, in addition to a role in mononuclear leukocyte recruitment through the vascular wall.

VIII. Selective Induction of VCAM-1 by Interleukin-4

The surface expression of ELAM-1, ICAM-1, and VCAM-1 on HUVECs *in vitro* is increased by the cytokines IL-1 and TNF, and by bacterial endotoxin (lipopolysaccharide), and these three proinflammatory mediators show little or no selectivity in their ability to induce adhesion molecule expression, at least *in vitro*. However, studies suggest that the cytokine interleukin-4 (IL-4) may show such selectivity (Masinovsky *et al.*, 1990; Thornhill *et al.*, 1990). Gallatin and co-workers were the first to show an effect of IL-4 on endothelial–leukocyte adhesion (Masinovksy *et al.*, 1990).

They examined the responses of cultured microvascular endothelial cells derived from macaque lymph nodes to various cytokines and found that markedly increased lymphocyte adhesion occurred after IL-4 treatment. Moreover, strong synergism with IL-1 for lymphocyte adhesion was observed. To identify the adhesion molecule responsible for these results, mAbs were generated that were selective for IL-4 treated endothelium, and one of these, 6G10, blocked up to 90% of lymphocyte adhesion to IL-4 treated cells. Subsequently, 6G10 was found to bind to CHO cells expressing human VCAM-1. The results indicated that macaque VCAM-1 was largely responsible for the observed lymphocyte adhesion, and more importantly, that VCAM-1 could be induced in endothelium by IL-4 (Masinovksy *et al.*, 1990).

In parallel studies using HUVECs, Haskard and co-workers found that IL-4 increased the adhesion of T-cells, but not PMN, to endothelium by inducing an adhesion pathway that was ICAM/LFA-1 independent (Thornhill *et al.*, 1990). They subsequently showed that IL-4 regulates endothelial cell activation by other cytokines (Thornhill and Haskard, 1990). In particular, IL-4 suppressed IL-1 or TNF induction of both ELAM-1 and ICAM-1, yet synergized with either cytokine for the induction of the antigen defined by mAb 1.4C3, later identified as VCAM-1 (Thornhill *et al.*, 1991).

The results suggest that IL-4 is unique in its ability to selectively modulate endothelial cell adhesion molecule expression. Its secretion by lymphocytes recruited to sites of inflammation or immune reactivity may serve to modulate local leukocyte accumulation, enhancing the transition from PMN rich to mononuclear leukocyte rich infiltrates during the evolution of inflammatory reactions.

IX. Summary

In summary, VCAM-1 is a member of the Ig superfamily that serves as an adhesion molecule, binding to the leukocyte integrin VLA-4. VCAM-1 was initially characterized by direct expression cloning techniques; independent studies in a number of laboratories generated mAbs found to recognize VCAM-1 on cytokine stimulated endothelium. These mAbs show not only that VCAM-1 is expressed on the vasculature at inflammatory sites where mononuclear leukocyte emigration is occurring, but also that VCAM-1 is constitutively expressed on dendritic and macrophage-like cells in normal tissues, supporting a role for VCAM-1 in the immune response as well as in leukocyte recruitment. In this regard, the VCAM-

1/VLA-4 interaction may well parallel the more extensively studied ICAM-1/LFA-1 interaction, also between members of the Ig and integrin superfamilies. The role of VCAM-1 in various pathologies in which mononuclear leukocyte accumulation is believed to play a role, such as allograft rejection, atherosclerosis, psoriasis, rheumatoid arthritis, and a variety of other autoimmune disorders, awaits the results of *in vivo* experiments.

Acknowledgments

We thank Drs. D. Briscoe, T. Carlos, V. Dixit, A. Koch, D. Haskard, J. Harlan, and B. Nickoloff for access to information either unpublished or in press.

References

Anderson, D. C., and Springer, T. A. (1987). *Annu. Rev. Med.* **38**, 175–194.

Beatty, P. G., Leadbetter, J. A., Martin, P. J., Price, T. H., and Hansen, J. A., (1983). *J. Immunol.***131**, 2913–2918.

Benjamin, C., Dougas, I., Chi-Rosso, G., Luhowskyj, S., Rosa, M., Newman, B., Osborn, L., Vassallo, C., Hession, C., Goelz, S., McCarthy, K., and Lobb, R. (1990). *Biochem. Biophys. Res. Commun.* **171**, 348–353.

Bevilacqua, M. P., and Gimbrone, M. A., Jr. (1989). *In* "Leukocyte Adhesion Molecules, Structure, Function, and Regulation" (T.A. Springer, D.C. Anderson, A.S. Rosenthal, and R. Rothlein, eds.), pp. 215–223. Springer-Verlag, New York.

Bevilacqua, M. P., Pober, J. S., Mendrick, D. L., Cotran, R. S., and Gimbrone, M. A., Jr. (1987). *Proc. Natl. Acad. Sci. U.S.A.* **84**, 9238–9242.

Bevilacqua, M. P., Stengelin, S., Gimbrone, M. A., Jr., and Seed, B. (1989). *Science* **243**, 1160–1165.

Brandley, B. K., Swiedler, S. J., and Robbins, P. W. (1990). *Cell* **63**, 861–863.

Briscoe, D. M., Schoen, F. J., Rice, G. E., Bevilacqua, M. P., Ganz, P., and Pober, J. S. (1991). *Transplantation* **51**, 537–547.

Carlos, T. M., Schwartz, B. R., Kovach, N. L., Yee, E., Rosa, M., Osborn, L., Chi-Rosso, G., Newman, B., Lobb, R., and Harlan, J. M. (1990). *Blood* **76**, 965–970.

Carlos, T. M., and Harlan, J. M. (1990). *Immunol. Rev.* **114**, 1–24.

Carlos, T., Kovach, N., Schwartz, B., Rosa, M., Newman, B., Wayner, E., Benjamin, C., Osborn, L., Lobb, R., and Harlan, J. (1991a). *Blood* **77**, 2266–2271.

Carlos, T., Gordon, D., Fishbein, D., Himes, V., Coday, A., Ross, R., and Allen, M. (1991b). *J. Heart Transplant.*(in press).

Cotran, R. S., and Pober, J. S. (1988). *In* "Endothelial Cell Biology" (N. Simionescu, and M. Simionescu, eds.), pp. 335–347. Plenum, New York.

Dejana, E., Bertocchi, F., Bortolami, M. C., Regonesi, A., Tonta, A., Brevario, F., and Giavazzi, R. (1988). *J. Clin. Invest.* **82**, 1466–1470.

Dustin, M. L., and Springer, T. A. (1988). *J. Cell. Biol.* **107**, 321–331.

Elices, M. J., Osborn, L., Takada, Y., Crouse, C., Luhowskyj, S., Hemler, M. E., and Lobb,

R. R. (1990). *Cell* **60**, 577–584.
Freedman, A. S., Munro, J. M., Rice, G. E., Bevilacqua, M. P., Morimoto, C., McIntyrem, B. W., Rhynhart, K., Pober, J. S., and Nadler, L. M. (1990). *Science* **249**, 1030–1033.
Graber, N., Gopal, T. V., Wilson, D., Beall, L. D., Polte, T., and Newman, W. (1990). *J. Immunol.* **145**, 819–830.
Griffiths, C. E. M., Barker, J. N. W. N., Kunkel, S., and Nickoloff, B. J. (1991). *Brit. J. Dermatol.* **124**, 519–526.
Harlan, J. M. (1985). *Blood* **65**, 513–525.
Haskard, D., Cavender, D., Beatty, P., Springer, T., and Ziff, M. (1986). *J. Immunol.* **137**, 2901–2906.
Hemler, M. E. (1990). *Annu. Rev. Immunol.* **8**, 365–400.
Hemperly, J. J., Murray, B. A., Edelman, G. M., and Cunningham, B. A. (1986). *Proc. Natl. Acad. Sci. U.S.A.* **83**, 3037–3041.
Hession, C., Osborn, L., Goff, D., Chi-Rosso, G., Vassallo, C., Pasek, M., Pittack, C., Tizard, R., Goelz, S., McCarthy, K., Hopple, S., and Lobb, R. (1990). *Proc. Natl. Acad. Sci. U.S.A.* **87**, 1673–1677.
Hession, C., Tizard, R., Vassallo, C., Schiffer, S. G., Goff, D., Moy, P., Chi-Rosso, G., Luhowskyj, S., Lobb, R., and Osborn, L. (1991). *J. Biol. Chem.* **266**, 6682–6685.
Hunkapillar, T., and Hood, L. (1989). *Adv. Immunol.* **44**, 1–63.
Hynes, R. O. (1987). *Cell* **48**, 549–554.
Kishimoto, T. K., Larson, R. S., Corbi, A. L., Dustin, M. L., Staunton, D. E., and Springer, T. A. (1989). *Adv. Immunol.* **46**, 149–182.
Koch, A. E., Burrows, J. C., Haines, K. G., Carlos, T., Harlan, J. M., and Leibovich, S. J. (1991). *Lab. Invest.* **64**, 313–320.
Lobb, R. R., Chi-Rosso, G., Leone, D., Rosa, M., Bixler, S., Newman, B., Luhowskyj, S., Benjamin, C., Dougas, I., Goelz, S., Hession, C., and Pingchang Chow, E. (1991). *J. Immunol.* **147**, 124–129.
Marcantonio, E. E., and Hynes, R. O. (1988). *J. Cell. Biol.* **106**, 1765–1772.
Marlin, S. D., and Springer, T. A. (1987). *Cell* **51**, 813–819.
Masinovsky, B., Urdal, D., and Gallatin, W. M. (1990). *J. Immunol.* **145**, 2886–2895.
Oikawa, S., Nakazato, H., and Kosaki, G. (1987). *Biochem. Biophys. Res. Commun.* **142**, 511–518.
Osborn, L. (1990). *Cell* **62**, 3–6.
Osborn, L., Hession, C., Tizard, R., Vassallo, C., Luhowskyj, S., Chi-Rosso, G., and Lobb, R. (1989). *Cell* **59**, 1203–1211.
Pober, J. S., and Cotran, R. S. (1990). *Transplantation* **50**, 537–544.
Pober, J. S., Gimbrone, M. A., Jr., Lapierre, L. A., Mendrick, D. L., Fiers, W., Rothlein, R., and Springer, T. A. (1986). *J. Immunol.* **137**, 1893–1896.
Polte, T., Newman, W., and Gopal, T. V. (1990). *Nucleic Acids Res.* **18**, 5901.
Rice, G. E., and Bevilacqua, M. P. (1989). *Science* **246**, 1303–1305.
Rice, G. E., Gimbrone, M. A., Jr., and Bevilacqua, M. P. (1988). *Am. J. Pathol.* **133**, 204–210.
Rice, G. E., Munro, J. M., and Bevilacqua, M. P. (1990). *J. Exp. Med.* **171**, 1369–1374.
Ruoslahti, E. (1988). *Annu. Rev. Biochem.* **57**, 375–413.
Schwartz, B. R., Wayner, E. A., Carlos, T. M., Ochs, H. D., and Harlan, J. M. (1990). *J. Clin. Invest.* **85**, 2019–2022.
Seed, B., and Aruffo, A. (1987). *Proc. Natl. Acad. Sci. U.S.A.* **84**, 3365–3369.
Simmons, D., Makgoba, M. W., and Seed, B. (1988). *Nature (London)* **331**, 624–627.
Springer, T. A. (1990). *Nature (London)* **346**, 425–434.
Staunton, D. E., Marlin, S. D., Stratowa, C., Dustin, M. L., and Springer, T. A. (1988). *Cell* **52**, 925–933.
Stoolman, L. M. (1989). *Cell* **56**, 907–910.

Thornhill, M. H., and Haskard, D. O. (1990). *J. Immunol.* **145**, 865–872.
Thornhill, M. H., Kyan-Aung, U., and Haskard, D. O. (1990). *J. Immunol.* **144**, 3060–3065.
Thornhill, M. H., Wellicome, S. M., Mahiouz, D. L., Lanchbury, J. S. S., Kyan-Aung, U., and Haskard, D. O. (1991). *J. Immunol.* **146,** 592–598.
Wayner, E. A., Garcia-Pardo, A., Humphries, M. J., McDonald, J. A., and Carter, W. G. (1989). *J. Cell. Biol.* **109**, 1321–1330.
Wellicome, S. M., Thornhill, M. H., Pitzalis, C., Thomas, D. S., Lanchberry, J. S. S., Panayi, G. S., and Haskard, D. O. (1990). *J. Immunol.* **144**, 2558–2565.
Williams, A. F., and Barclay, A. N. (1988). *Annu. Rev. Immunol.* **6**, 381–405.

CHAPTER 9

The Role of Intercellular Adhesion Molecule-1 (ICAM-1) in the Inflammatory Response

Robert Rothlein, Randall W. Barton, and Raymond Winquist

Boehringer Ingelheim Pharmaceuticals, Inc.
Ridgefield, Connecticut 06877

I. Leukocyte Adhesion in Inflammation: Role of CD18 Adhesion Molecules

Leukocyte–leukocyte and leukocyte–target cell adhesion is a mandatory process for the host defense system to perform normally in an inflammatory response. Leukocytes must attach to endothelial cells lining blood vessels prior to migrating from the circulation to inflamed lesions. For specific immunological processes, such as antibody production or the generation of antigen specific T-cells, to occur, lymphocytes must first attach to antigen presenting cells. Finally, for leukocytes to perform effector functions, such as lysis of target cells, they must first attach to these cells so that locally high concentrations of lytic mediators secreted by the leukocyte can be attained at the leukocyte–target cell junction.

Through two converging lines of evidence during the last 10 years, the CD18 family of molecules on leukocytes has been implicated as being partially responsible for mediating leukocyte adhesion to cellular substrates. The CD18 family, or LFA-1 family of adhesion molecules, consist of CD11a, CD18 (LFA-1), CD11b, CD18 (MAC-1), and CD11c, CD18 (p150,95) (reviewed in Springer *et al.*, 1987; Martz, 1987; Springer, 1990). These molecules are each heterodimers with distinct alpha subunits that associate with a common beta subunit. These molecules are distributed in various combinations on all leukocytes. Structurally, the leukocyte adhesion molecules are members of the integrin supergene family and specifically they belong to the β2 subgroup. Although the leukocyte adhesion molecules mediate adhesion processes, they are unlike most other integrins in that they appear to recognize ligands that, for the most part, do not contain RGD sequences, and their activity is dependent on Mg^{++}rather than Ca^{++} (Rothlein and Springer, 1986; Marlin and Springer, 1987).

The first line of evidence to show the function of these molecules, and indeed the importance of leukocyte adhesion in the generation and maintenance of inflammation, were elucidated in many experimental systems where mAb to these molecules were used as antagonists and found to inhibit multiple events associated with inflammation. *In vitro*, mAb to CD18 or CD11a inhibit lymphocyte mediated lytic events, such as cytotoxic T-cell activity and natural killer cell activity (Krensky *et al.*, 1983; Sanchez-Madrid *et al.*, 1983; Kohl *et al.*, 1984), and lymphocyte trafficking processes, such as attachment of lymphocytes to vascular endothelium and epidermal cells (Haskard *et al.*, 1986; Dustin *et al.*, 1988). Furthermore, these mAb inhibited antibody formation and mitogen and antigen induced T-cell proliferation as well as the mixed lymphocyte response (MLR) (Davignon *et al.*, 1981; Dougherty *et al.*, 1988; Dougherty and Hogg, 1987; Boyd *et al.*, 1988). All of these processes require cell–cell interaction for successful responses. mAb to CD18 and to CD11 also inhibit granulocyte function, such as attachment to endothelium (Smith *et al.*, 1988), homotypic aggregation (Anderson *et al.*, 1986), binding to iC3b coated particles (Beller *et al.*, 1982; Anderson *et al.*, 1986), and antibody dependent cellular cytotoxicity (Kohl *et al.*, 1984).

The second line of evidence that suggested an important role of the CD18 family of adhesion molecules came from the identification of a group of individuals who, due to genetic defects, were unable to express the normal number of leukocyte adhesion molecules on their cell surfaces (Anderson and Springer, 1987; Todd and Freyer, 1988). These patients were classified into a *severely deficient group* (expressing between 0 to 1% of the normal number of adhesion molecules on the leukocyte surface) and a *moderately deficient group* (expressing between 2 to 10% of the normal number of adhesion molecules on the leukocyte surface) (Anderson *et al.*, 1985). Both groups of individuals presented with delayed umbilical cord separation, frequent skin infections with little leukocyte infiltrate, and no pus formation. The severely deficient patients had depressed T-cell responses also, presumably because of defective antigen presenting capacity caused by the inability of the T-cell to attach to the antigen presenting cell. *In vitro*, lymphocytes from these individuals behaved as did normal lymphocytes in the presence of anti-LFA-1 mAb. They had defective proliferative and effector responses in assays requiring cell–cell interactions (Mentzer *et al.*, 1986).

II. Intercellular Adhesion Molecule-1 (ICAM-1): A CD18 Ligand

A. Functional Characterization

A ligand of LFA-1 is intercellular adhesion molecule-1 (ICAM-1), which was functionally identified by screening antibodies from hybridomas generated from spleen cells of mice immunized against LFA-1 deficient lymphocytes for their ability to inhibit an LFA-1 dependent homotypic adhesion assay (Rothlein and Springer, 1986; Rothlein *et al.*, 1986). One antibody was identified, and it was subsequently shown that the antigen that was affinity purified using this antibody, when inserted into planar membranes or immobilized on plastic, was able to mediate lymphocyte adhesion (Marlin and Springer, 1987; Makgoba *et al.*, 1988). This adhesion was inhibitable by mAb directed against either ICAM-1 or LFA-1. Thus, it was clear that ICAM-1 was a counterstructure for LFA-1.

What was not clear until several years later was that ICAM-1 also mediated neutrophil adhesion to endothelium and that ICAM-1 was a ligand for MAC-1. These data came from several sources. Firstly, in several papers Smith *et al.* (1989) showed that a mouse IgG2a monoclonal anti-ICAM-1 antibody, R6.5, inhibited the attachment of neutrophils to endothelial cells to the same extent that an anti-CD18 monoclonal antibody did. This suggested that ICAM-1 played a role in neutrophil adhesion to endothelium (Smith *et al.*, 1988). They then showed that neutrophils adhered to ICAM-1 in planar membranes and that this adhesion was inhibited by anti-CD18 binding to neutrophils and by anti-ICAM-1 binding to the planar membrane. Furthermore, all neutrophil adhesion to ICAM-1 containing planar membranes was inhibited by anti-CD11a antibodies when the neutrophils were not exposed to chemotactic stimuli. However, stimulated neutrophil adhesion to ICAM-1 in planar membranes was only partially inhibited by anti-CD11a and partially inhibited by anti-CD11b. The combination of both antibodies inhibited neutrophil adhesion to ICAM-1 in planar membranes to the same extent as anti-CD18 or anti-ICAM-1 (Smith *et al.*, 1989). These data imply that LFA-1 on unactivated neutrophils are the only adhesion molecules capable of binding to ICAM-1. However, when the neutrophil becomes activated, MAC-1 also binds to ICAM-1. Whether the newly expressed MAC-1 on activated neutrophils are the only MAC-1 molecules capable of binding to ICAM-1 or whether activation modifies, modulates, or both constitutively expressed MAC-1 to mediate ICAM-1 dependent adhesion is not clear. That MAC-1 binds to ICAM-1 was subsequently confirmed by Diamond *et al.* in a series of experiments showing that ICAM-1 transfected COS cells and L-cells adhered to immobilized purified MAC-1, and MAC-1 transfected COS cells adhered to immobilized purified ICAM-1 (Diamond *et al.*, 1989; Diamond *et al.*, 1990). All of these adhesion systems were inhibited by appropriate anti-ICAM-1 or anti-CD11/CD18 antibodies. Furthermore, it was concluded that while LFA-1 and MAC-1 both bind to ICAM-1, their sites of interaction on the ICAM-1 molecule are probably distinct because different anti-ICAM-1 antibodies have differential inhibitory effects on LFA-1/ICAM-1 versus MAC-1/ICAM-1 interactions.

B. Structure of ICAM-1

Structurally, ICAM-1 is a member of the immunoglobulin supergene family with five Ig-like domains, a single membrane spanning region, and a short cytoplasmic tail (Staunton *et al.*, 1988; Simmons *et al.*, 1988). It has also been shown to bind the major rhinoviruses (Greve *et al.*, 1989; Diamond *et al.*, 1990). Staunton *et al.*, using domain deletion and site directed mutagenesis, has clearly distinguished between the site of ICAM-1 that binds to LFA-1 and the rhinovirus binding site. As deduced from chimeric molecules between human domains 1 and 2 expressed on mouse domains 3 to 5 and mouse domains 1 and 2 on human domains 3 to 5, binding activity for both LFA-1 and human rhinovirus 14 resides on domains 1 and 2 of ICAM-1. Furthermore, three anti-ICAM-1 antibodies that are known to functionally interfere with LFA-1/ICAM-1 interactions also map to domains 1 and 2 of ICAM-1 (Staunton *et al.*, 1990).

C. Expression of ICAM-1

Further characterization of ICAM-1 revealed that it was induced *in vitro* on multiple cell types including hematopoietic cells, endothelial cells, and fibroblasts with IL-1α, IL-1β, TNF-α, TNF-β, IFN-gamma, or all of these depending on the cell type (Dustin *et al.*, 1986; Dustin *et al.*, 1988; Pober *et al.*, 1986; Frohman *et al.*, 1989). Functionally, anti-ICAM-1 mAb inhibited *in vitro* assays, such as MLRs (Boyd *et al.*, 1988), antigen induced proliferation (Dougherty *et al.*, 1988), cytotoxic T-cell activity (Mentzer *et al.*, 1988; Makgoba *et al.*, 1989), and granulocyte and lymphocyte attachment to endothelium (Smith *et al.*, 1988; Smith *et al.*, 1989; Dustin and Springer, 1988). Furthermore, when ICAM-1 was transfected into L-cells expressing low amounts of HLA-DR molecules, enhanced class II restricted proliferation was attained when compared to L-cells expressing the HLA-DR alone (Altmann *et al.*, 1989), and ICAM-1 defective mutants were unable to properly present antigen to mouse T-cells (Dang *et al.*, 1990). These data suggested that, like the CD18 family of adhesion molecules, ICAM-1 expression on endothelial cells and other cell types was critical for the normal function of the host defense system.

Equally as suggestive is the expression of ICAM-1 at sites of inflammation. There is a low constitutive expression of ICAM-1 on venule endothelial cells, and its expression is markedly increased at inflammatory sites (Dustin *et al.*, 1986). Furthermore, there is an increased ICAM-1 expression on multiple cell types including keratinocytes in inflamed skin lesions (Vejlsgaard *et al.*, 1989; Griffiths and Nickoloff, 1989), transplanted liver bile duct (Adams *et al.*, 1989) and perivenular hepatocytes during rejection, endothelium in the brain surrounding MS plaques and EAE lesions in man and rodent, respectively (Sobel *et al.*, 1990; Frohman *et al.*, 1989; Raine *et al.*, 1990a, b; Cannella *et al.*, 1990; Wilcox *et al.*, 1990), transplanted kidney glomeruli and tubules during rejection (Cosimi *et al.*, 1990), as well as lung epithelial cells following antigen provocation (Wegner *et al.*, 1990). Increased ICAM-1 is also found on melanoma cells following metastasis (Matsui *et al.*, 1987; Natali *et al.*, 1990).

III. *In Vivo* Activity of Anti-ICAM-1 Monoclonal Antibodies

A. Inflammatory Models

The *in vivo* activity of anti-ICAM-1 mAb has been assessed in several animal models of inflammation. Anti-ICAM-1 mAb has been shown to inhibit neutrophil influx into rabbit lungs following systemic activation with phorbol esters (Barton *et al.*, 1989). Furthermore, anti-ICAM-1 mAb mitigated eosinophil influx and airway hyperresponsiveness in a nonhuman primate model of antigen induced airway hyperresponsiveness (Wegner *et al.*, 1990). Finally, it was reported that anti-ICAM-1, when given to nonhuman primates daily for 12 days, more than doubled the survival time of kidney allografts from an average of less than 10 days in the untreated animals to greater than 22 days in the treated animals (Cosimi *et al.*, 1990). Furthermore, anti-ICAM-1 mAb reversed acute rejection episodes in monkeys given suboptimal doses of cyclosporin A. Of interest in the latter study, biopsies from monkeys receiving anti-ICAM-1 still revealed a heavy leukocyte infiltrate even though biochemical parameters of kidney rejection, such as serum creatinine levels, were normal. This suggests that one mode of action of the anti-ICAM-1 mAb was to inhibit leukocyte–target cell conjugation rather than solely inhibiting leukocyte trafficking. Alternatively, inhibition of LFA-1/ICAM-1 interactions may prevent necessary cosignalling as has been previously described (Wacholtz *et al.*, 1989; Van Seventer *et al.*, 1990).

B. Shwartzman Reaction

We found that anti-ICAM-1 mAb was effective in inhibiting several new models of neutrophil mediated inflammation. The local Shwartzman reaction can be produced in rabbit skin by an *i.d.* injection of endotoxin followed by an *i.v.* challenge injection of zymosan 18 to 24 hours later (Argenbright and Barton, 1991). An inflammatory response develops only in the skin sites that were previously injected with endotoxin and is directly endotoxin dose dependent. The inflammation is characterized by intravascular neutrophil aggregation, increased vascular permeability, platelet aggregation, fibrin deposition, and hemorrhage (Movat *et al.*, 1980). Quantitation of the microvascular hemorrhage using ^{99}mTc labeled RBCs showed a 5-fold increase in RBCs in endotoxin injected sites 3 hours after systemic challenge. As shown in Table I, administration of anti-ICAM-1 only prior to the systemic challenge was effective in inhibiting hemorrhage. Similar inhibition of hemorrhage was seen when anti-CD18 was injected prior to challenge.

These results indicate that the Shwartzman response is a CD18/ICAM-1 dependent inflammatory response. The marked inhibitory effect of the anti-ICAM-1 suggests that ICAM-1 was up-regulated by the preparatory injection of endotoxin. Endotoxin, IL-1β, and TNF-α are effective for preparative injections in the Shwartzman reaction (Movat *et al.*, 1987), and all of these molecules are known to up-regulate ICAM-1 on endothelial cells

TABLE I

Inhibition of Hemorrhage in the Shwartzman Reaction by Anti-CD18/ICAM-1 Monoclonal Antibodies

Antibody	% of control
Control mouse Ig	94 ± 5
Anti-ICAM-1	18 ± 7
Anti-CD18	10 ± 5

in vitro (Pober *et al.*, 1986; Pohlman *et al.*, 1986). In contrast, neutrophil chemotactic factors, such as fMLP and C5a, cannot function as preparatory agents (Fehr *et al.*, 1984) and do not up-regulate ICAM-1. These findings suggest that the requirement for a preparative agent in the Shwartzman reaction is the induction of expression of ICAM-1.

Unlike some models of vasculitis, the Shwartzman reaction is not immune complex mediated. However, the inflammation that is seen in the Shwartzman reaction may proceed by pathways common to many clinical conditions. Examples of these include disseminated intravascular coagulation, systemic lupus erythematosus, adult respiratory distress syndrome, and myocardial infarction.

C. Myocardial Ischemia/Reperfusion

Prompted by the realization that myocardial infarction has many similarities to an acute inflammatory response, several studies were successful in demonstrating beneficial effects of treatments aimed at diminishing leukocyte count or function in models of cardiac ischemia or reperfusion injury [e.g. (Romson *et al.*, 1983; Simpson and Lucchesi, 1987)]. The role of ICAM-1 in mediating the detrimental effects of leukocytes in these models had been assessed by administering the anti-ICAM-1 mAb (R6.5) prior to the ischemic event. R6.5 (1 mg/kg, *i.v.*) was found to provide protection against the development of myocardial necrosis in a rabbit model of 60 minutes occlusion followed by 5 hours of reperfusion (Seewaldt-Becker *et al.*, 1990). Administration of the mAb 15 minutes prior to the ischemic event reduced infarct size by 51% compared to saline treated controls. A nonspecific murine mAb was without any significant effect.

We have conducted preliminary experiments using R6.5 in a primate model of myocardial ischemia/reperfusion injury (Fig. 1). Anesthetized monkeys treated with R6.5 (1 mg/kg, *i.v.*) 30 minutes prior to 90 minutes

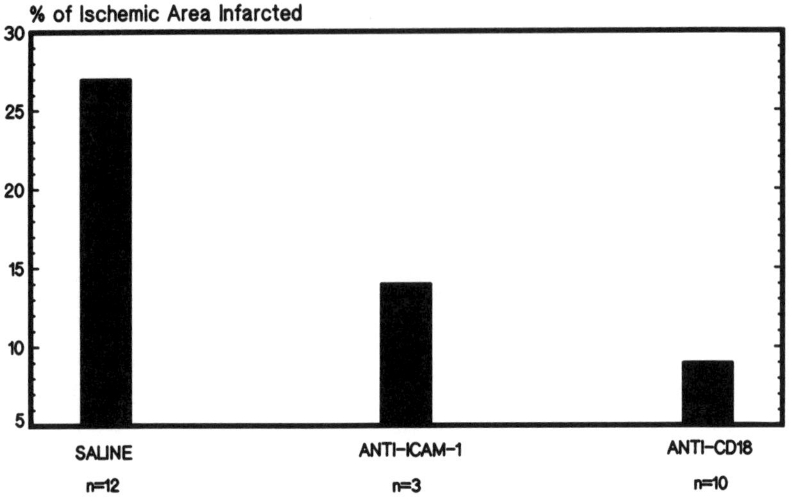

FIGURE 1

Reduction of myocardial infarct size by anti-ICAM-1. Studies in anesthetized cynomolgus monkeys.

of ischemia and 4 hours of reperfusion had less myocardial necrosis compared to a saline treated control group. It is of interest to note that the efficacy of the anti-ICAM-1 mAb in these two models was similar to that obtained with a mAb directed against CD18. Therefore, ICAM-1 associated adhesion pathways appear important in the trafficking of, and possibly the release of lytic mediators from activated leukocytes during myocardial ischemia or reperfusion injury.

These data show the critical importance of the leukocyte adhesion molecules and ICAM-1 in the inflammatory response and suggest that interfering with the interaction of the CD18 molecules with ICAM-1 offer a promising new target for anti-inflammatory drug development.

References

Adams, D. H., Hubscher, S. G., Shaw, J., Rothlein, R., and Neuberger, J. M. (1989). *Lancet* **2**, 1122.

Altmann, D. M., Hogg, N., Trowsdale, J., and Wilkinson, D. (1989). *Nature (London)* **338**, 512.

Anderson, D. C., Miller, L. J., Schmalstieg, F. C., Rothlein, R., and Springer, T. A. (1986). *J. Immunol.* **137**, 15.

Anderson, D. C., Schmalstieg, F. C., Finegold, M. J., Hughes, B. J., Rothlein, R., Miller, L. J., Kohl, S., Tosi, M. F., Jacobs, R. L., Waldrop, T. C., Goldman, A. S., Shearer, W. T., and Springer, T. A. (1985). *J. Inf. Dis.* **152**, 668.

Anderson, D. C., and Springer, T. A. (1987). *Ann. Rev. Med.* **38**, 175.

Argenbright, L. W., and Barton, R. (1991). *Agents and Actions* (in press).

Barton, R. W., Rothlein, R., Ksiazek, J., and Kennedy, C. (1989). *J. Immunol.* **143**, 1278.

Beller, D. I., Springer, T. A., and Schreiber, R. D. (1982). *J. Exp. Med.* **156**, 1000.

Boyd, A. W., Wawryk, S. O., Burns, G. F., and Fecondo, J. V. (1988). *Proc. Natl. Acad. Sci. U.S.A.* **85**, 3095.

Cannella, B., Cross, A. H., and Raine, C. S. (1990). *J. Exp. Med.* **172**, 1521.

Cosimi, A. B., Conti, D., Delmonico, F. L., Preffer, F. I., Wee, S.-L., Rothlein, R., Faanes, R., and Colvin, R. B. (1990). *J. Immunol.* **144**, 4604.

Dang, L. H., Michalek, M. T., Takei, F., Benaceraff, B., and Rock, K. L. (1990). *J. Immunol.* **144**, 4082.

Davignon, D., Martz, E., Reynolds, T., Kührzinger, K., and Springer, T. A. (1981). *J. Immunol.* **127**, 590.

Diamond, M. S., McCaffery, P., Johnston, S. C., Dustin, M., and Springer, T. A. (1989). *In* "Leukocyte Typing IV," pp. 570–574. Oxford Press, New York.

Diamond, M. S., Staunton, D. E., De Fougerolles, A. R., Stacker, S. A., Garcia-Aguilar, J., Hibbs, M. L., and Springer, T. A. (1990). *J. Cell. Biol.* **111**, 3129.

Dougherty, G. J., and Hogg, N. (1987). *Eur. J. Immunol.* **17**, 943.

Dougherty, G. J., Murdoch, S., and Hogg, N. (1988). *Eur. J. Immunol.* **18**, 35.

Dustin, M. L., and Springer, T. A. (1988). *J. Cell. Biol.* **107**, 321.

Dustin, M. L., Rothlein, R., Bhan, A. K., Dinarello, C. A., and Springer, T. A. (1986). *J. Immunol.* **137**, 245.

Dustin, M. L., Singer, K. H., Tuck, D. T., and Springer, T. A. (1988). *J. Exp. Med.* **167**, 1323.

Fehr, R. T., Dahinden, C., and Russi, R. (1984). *J. Infect. Dis.* **150**, 160.

Frohman, E. M., Frohman, T. C., Dustin, M. L., Vayuvegula, B., Choi, B., Gupta, A., van den Noort, S., and Gupta, S. (1989). *J. Neuroimmunol.* **23**, 117.

Greve, J. M., Davis, G., Meyer, A. M., Forte, C. P., Yost, S. C., Marlor, C. W., Kamarck, M. E., and McClelland, A. (1989). *Cell* **56**, 839.

Griffiths, C. E. M., and Nickoloff, B. J. (1989). *Am. J. Pathol.* **135**, 1045.

Haskard, D., Cavender, D., Beatty, P., Springer, T. A., and Ziff, M. (1986). *J. Immunol.* **137**, 2901.

Kohl, S., Springer, T. A., Schmalstieg, F. C., Loo, L. S., and Anderson, D. C. (1984). *J. Immunol.* **133**, 2972.

Krensky, A. M., Sanchez-Madrid, F., Robbins, E., Nagy, J., Springer, T. A., and Burakoff, S. J. (1983). *J. Immunol.* **131**, 611.

Makgoba, M. W., Sanders, M. E., Luce, G. E. G., Dustin, M. L., Springer, T. A., Clark, E. A., Mannoni, P., and Shaw, S. (1988). *Nature (London)* **331**, 86.

Makgoba, M. W., Sanders, M. E., Luce, G. E. G., Gugel, E. A., Dustin, M. L., Springer, T. A., and Shaw, S. (1989). *Ann. N.Y. Acad. Sci.* **532**, 427.

Marlin, S. D., and Springer, T. A. (1987). *Cell* **51**, 813.

Martz, E. (1987). *Human Immunol.* **18**, 3.

Matsui, M., Temponi, M., and Ferrone, S. (1987). *J. Immunol.* **139**, 2088.

Mentzer, S. J., Bierer, B. E., Anderson, D. C., Springer, T. A., and Burakoff, S. J. (1986). *J. Clin. Invest.* **78**, 1387.

Mentzer, S. J., Rothlein, R., Springer, T. A., and Faller, D. V. (1988). *J. Cell. Physiol.* **137**, 173.

Movat, H. Z., Jaynes, B. J., Wasi, S., Movat, K. W., and Kopaniak, M. M. (1980). *In* "Bacterial Endotoxins and Host Response" (M. K. Agarwal, ed.), pp. 179–201. Elsevier, Amsterdam.

Movat, H. Z., Burrows, C. E., Cybulsky, M. I., and Dinarello, C. A. (1987). *Am. J. Pathol.* **129**, 463.

Natali, P., Nicotra, M. R., Cavaliere, R., Bigotti, A., Romano, G., Temponi, M., and Ferrone, S. (1990). *Cancer Res.* **50**, 1271.

Pober, J. S., Gimbrone, M. A., Jr., Lapierre, L. A., Mendrick, D. L., Fiers, W., Rothlein, R., and Springer, T. A. (1986). *J. Immunol.* **137**, 1893.

Pohlman, T. H., Stanness, K. A., Beatty, P. G., Ochs, H. D., and Harlan, J. M. (1986). *J. Immunol.* **136**, 4548.

Raine, C. S., Cannella, B., Duijvestijn, A. M., and Cross, A. H. (1990a). *Lab. Invest.* **63**, 476.

Raine, C. S., Lee, S. C., Scheinberg, L. C., Duijvestijn, A. M., and Cross, A. H. (1990b). *Clin. Immunol. Immunopathol.* **57**, 173.

Romson, J. L., Hook, B. G., Kunkel, S. L., Abrams, G. D., Schork, M. A., and Lucchesi, B. R. (1983). *Circulation* **67**, 1016.

Rothlein, R., Dustin, M. L., Marlin, S. D., and Springer, T. A. (1986). *J. Immunol.* **137**, 1270.

Rothlein, R., and Springer, T. A. (1986). *J. Exp. Med.* **163**, 1132.

Sanchez-Madrid, F., Nagy, J., Robbins, E., Simon, P., and Springer, T. A. (1983). *J. Exp. Med.* **158**, 1785.

Seewaldt-Becker, E., Rothlein, R., and Dammgen, J. (1990). *In* "Leukocyte Adhesion Molecules: Structure, Function, and Regulation" (T. A. Springer, D. C. Anderson, A. S. Rosenthal, and R. Rothlein, eds.), pp. 138–148. Springer-Verlag, New York.

Simmons, D., Makgoba, M. W., and Seed, B. (1988). *Nature (London)* **331**, 624.

Simpson, P. J., and Lucchesi, B. R. (1987). *J. Lab. Clin. Med.* **110**, 13.

Smith, C. W., Rothlein, R., Hughes, B. J., Mariscalco, M. M., Schmalstieg, F. C., and Anderson, D. C. (1988). *J. Clin. Invest.* **82**, 1746.

Smith, C. W., Marlin, S. D., Rothlein, R., Toman, C., and Anderson, D. C. (1989). *J. Clin. Invest.* **83**, 2008.

Sobel, R. A., Mitchell, M. E., and Fondren, G. (1990). *Am. J. Pathol.* **136**, 1309.

Springer, T. A. (1990). *Nature (London)* **346**, 425.

Springer, T. A., Dustin, M. L., Kishimoto, T. K., and Marlin, S. D. (1987). *Ann. Rev. Immunol.* **5**, 223.

Staunton, D. E., Dustin, M. L., Erickson, H. P., and Springer, T. A. (1990). *Cell* **61**, 243.

Staunton, D. E., Marlin, S. D., Stratowa, C., Dustin, M. L., and Springer, T. A. (1988). *Cell* **52**, 925.

Todd, R. F., and Freyer, D. R. (1988). *Hem./Onc. Clinics N.A.* **2**, 13.

Van Seventer, G. A., Shimizu, Y., Horgan, K. J., and Shaw, S. (1990). *J. Immunol.* **144**, 4579.

Vejlsgaard, G. L., Ralfkiaer, E., Avnstorp, C., Czajkowski, M., Marlin, S. D., and Rothlein, R. (1989). *J. Am. Acad. Dermtol.* **20**, 782.

Wacholtz, M. C., Patel, S. S., and Lipsky, P. E. (1989). *J. Exp. Med.* **170**, 431.

Wegner, C. D., Gundel, R. H., Reilly, P., Haynes, N., Letts, L. G., and Rothlein, R. (1990). *Science* **247**, 456.

Wilcox, C. E., Ward, A. M. V., Evans, A., Baker, D., Rothlein, R., and Turk, J. L. (1990). *J. Neuroimmunol.* **30**, 43.

Index